Welcome!

I'll Cook, You Color is a unique and delightful coloring cookbook that brings together the joy of cooking and the creativity of coloring. Inside, you'll find delicious recipes paired with beautifully illustrated pages to color, making it a perfect blend of culinary inspiration and artistic expression. Whether you're a seasoned chef or a budding artist, this book offers a fun and relaxing way to explore new recipes while adding your personal touch to each page. Unleash your inner chef and artist with **I'll Cook, You Color**!

To our family and friends, whose endless support and love have been the ingredients of our success; this book is for you. May it add color to your kitchens and joy to your hearts, just as you have done for us.

Jai Lee

www.designedbyjai.com

Food Disclaimer

The recipes provided in this book are for informational purposes only and are intended to offer a general guide to cooking. While we strive to ensure all recipes are accurate and safe, we cannot guarantee that the instructions will suit every individual's needs or circumstances; so feel free to tweak them to your liking.

Important Considerations:

1. Allergies and Dietary Restrictions:
• Always check the ingredients for potential allergens before preparing any recipe. If you have specific dietary restrictions or allergies, substitute ingredients accordingly.

2. Food Safety:
• Follow standard food safety practices. Ensure all meats are cooked to the appropriate temperatures, and all fruits and vegetables are washed thoroughly before use.
• Avoid cross-contamination by using separate utensils and cutting boards for raw and cooked foods. Also, be sure to wash your hands and maintain a clean working area.

3. Nutritional Information:
• Nutritional values provided are estimates and can vary based on quantity and quality. For precise dietary advice, consult a registered dietitian or nutritionist.

4. Health Concerns:
• Consult with your healthcare provider before making significant changes to your diet, especially if you have any underlying health conditions.

The authors and publishers of this book are not responsible for any adverse reactions, effects, or health issues resulting from the use of recipes or ingredients mentioned in this book. Use these recipes at your own risk and discretion.

Safety Note

While this cookbook is designed to be a fun and educational experience for all ages, it's important to prioritize safety in the kitchen.

For Parents and Guardians:

Please ensure that children under the age of 12 do not use sharp kitchen tools, such as knives or graters, or operate stoves and ovens without adult supervision. Always provide guidance and assistance to young cooks to ensure a safe and enjoyable cooking experience. Thank you for helping to create a safe and happy kitchen environment!

all about me

My name is: _____

My age is: _____

My favorite color is: _____

I am from: _____

My birthday is: _____

This is me

My favorite fruits are:	My favorite vegetables are:

My favorite food is:	My wish for this year is:

TABLE OF CONTENTS

Strawberries

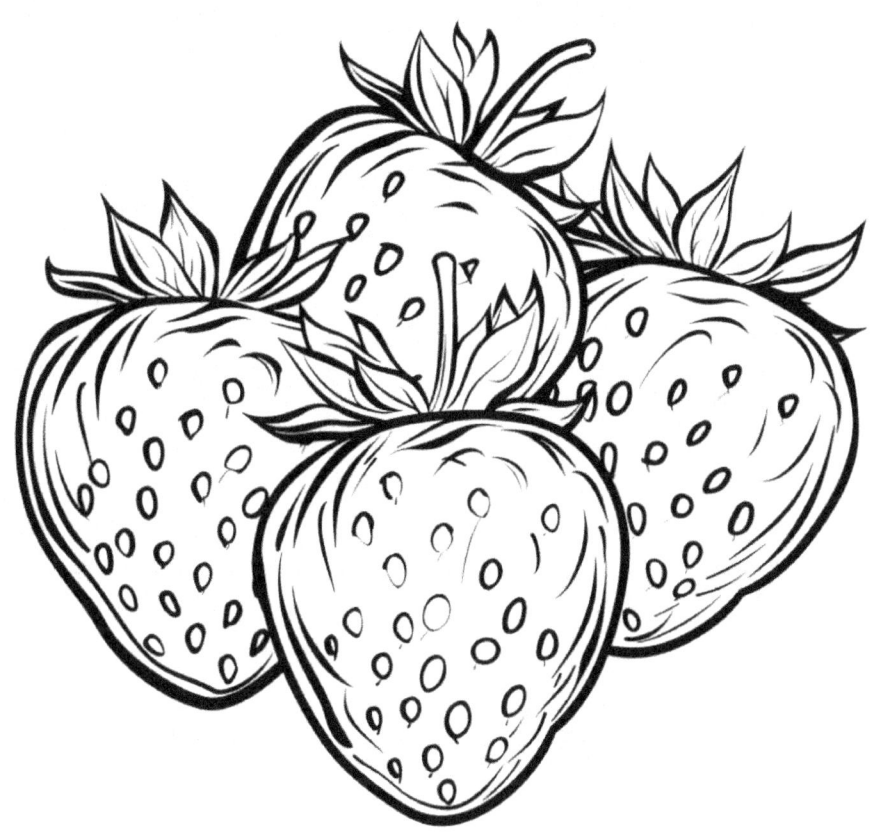

NUTRITION FACTS

Rich in Antioxidants
Strawberries contain high levels of antioxidants like vitamin C, manganese, and various polyphenols, which help combat oxidative stress and inflammation in the body.

Heart Health
Strawberries are beneficial for heart health. They help lower blood pressure, reduce cholesterol levels, and improve the function of blood vessels. The high fiber, potassium, and antioxidant content contribute to these cardiovascular benefits.

Immune Support
Studies indicate strawberries help the body fight off infections and illnesses effectively due to the high vitamin C content.

Strawberries are also good for:
- Blood Sugar Regulation
- Skin Health
- Digestive Health
- Cancer Prevention
- Weight Management
- Eye Health

Step-by-Step Cleaning Instructions

1. Sort the strawberries by removing bruised, moldy, or damaged strawberries.
2. Rinse thoroughly under cold running water using a colander.
3. Use a Vinegar Solution for Extra Cleanliness: In a large bowl, mix one-part white vinegar with three parts water. Place the strawberries in the vinegar solution and let them soak for about 5 minutes. This helps to remove more pesticides and bacteria.
4. Rinse strawberries under cold running water after soaking them.
5. Dry the strawberries by laying them out on a clean kitchen towel and pat them dry gently with another towel or paper towel.

Strawberry Overnight Oats

- 1/2 cup rolled oats
- 1/2 cup milk (or almond milk)
- 1/4 cup Greek yogurt
- 1 tablespoon chia seeds
- 1 tablespoon honey
- 1/2 cup frozen or fresh strawberries

1. In a mason jar or container, combine oats, milk, Greek yogurt, chia seeds, and honey.
2. Stir in the strawberries.
3. Cover and refrigerate overnight.
4. In the morning, stir the oats and enjoy cold or warmed up.

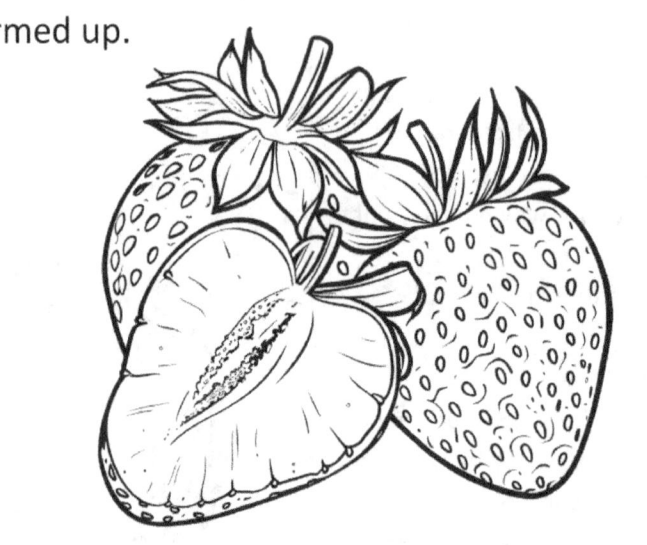

Strawberry Smoothie

- 1 cup frozen/fresh strawberries
- 1 banana
- 1 cup milk (or almond milk)
- 1/2 cup Greek yogurt
- 1 tablespoon honey (optional)

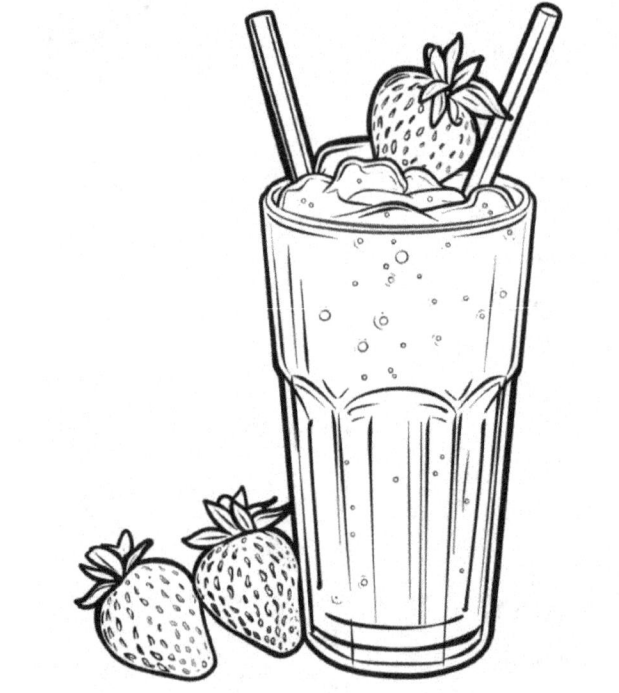

1. Add all ingredients to a blender.
2. Blend until smooth.
3. Pour into a glass and enjoy immediately.

Strawberry Sorbet

- 4 cups frozen/fresh strawberries
- 1/2 cup sugar
- 1/4 cup water
- 1 tablespoon lemon juice

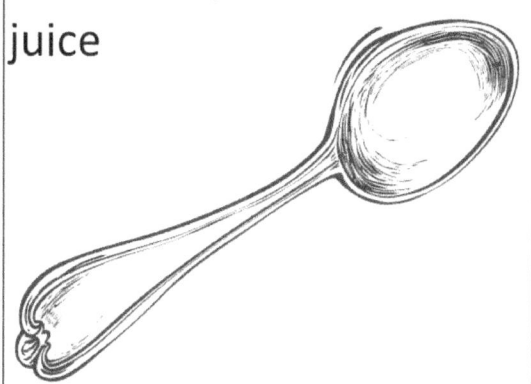

1. In a small saucepan, combine sugar and water. Heat until sugar dissolves, then let cool.
2. In a blender, blend the strawberries until smooth.
3. Add the sugar and lemon juice to the strawberries and blend until well combined.
4. Transfer the mixture to a container and freeze for at least 2 hours before serving.

Strawberry Breakfast Bars

- 1 ½ cups rolled oats
- ½ cup almond flour
- ¼ cup honey or maple syrup
- ¼ cup coconut oil, melted
- 1 tsp vanilla extract
- 1 cup fresh strawberries, chopped
- 1 tbsp chia seeds

1. Preheat oven to 350°F (175°C). Line an 8x8-inch baking dish with parchment paper.
2. In a large bowl, mix together oats, almond flour, honey, coconut oil, and vanilla extract.
3. Fold in the chopped strawberries and chia seeds.
4. Press the mixture evenly into the prepared baking dish.
5. Bake for 20-25 minutes or until golden brown.
6. Let cool completely before cutting into bars.

Blueberries

NUTRITION FACTS

Weight Management
Blueberries are low in calories and high in fiber, making them a nutrient dense snack that can aid in weight management.

Improved Brain Function
Regular consumption of blueberries has been linked to improved cognitive function and memory due to their high antioxidant content.

Blood Sugar Control
The fiber in blueberries helps regulate blood sugar levels, making them a good choice for diabetes prevention.

Blueberries Contain:
- **Vitamin C**
- **Vitamin K**
- **Vitamin E**
- **Vitamin B6**
- **Folate**
- **Potassium**
- **Manganese**
- **Copper**
- **Iron**

1 Cup (Approx. 148g) of Blueberries Contain:
- Calories: 84
- Protein: 1.1 grams
- Fat: 0.5 grams
- Carbs: 21.4 grams
- Fiber: 3.6 grams
- Sugars: 14.7 grams

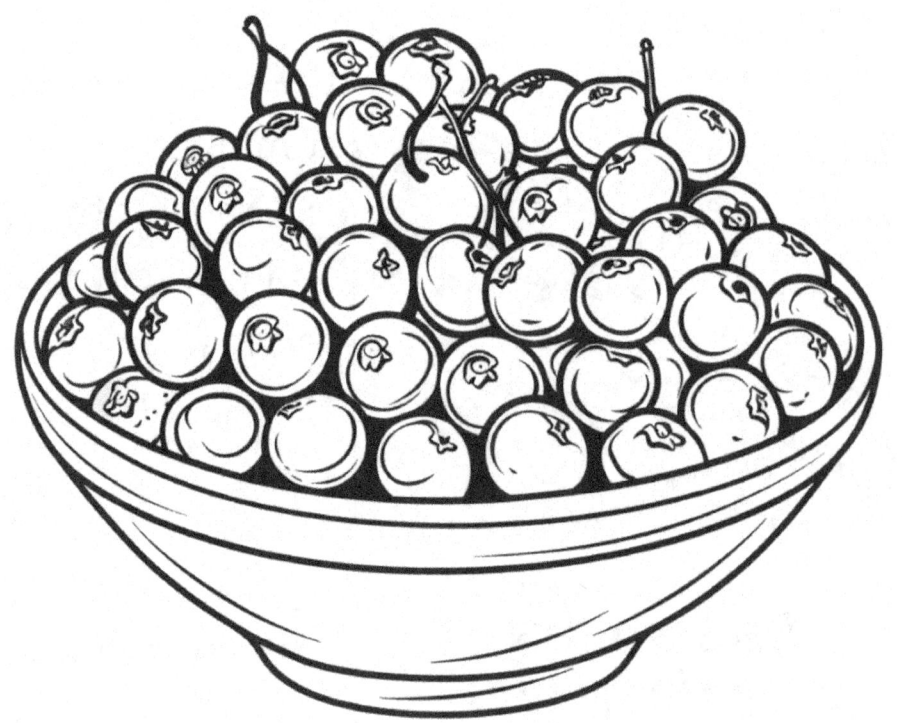

Step-by-Step Cleaning Instructions

- Sort the blueberries by removing the bruised, moldy, or damaged ones.
- Rinse thoroughly under cold running water using a colander.
- Use a Vinegar Solution for Extra Cleanliness: In a large bowl, mix one-part white vinegar with three parts water. Place the blueberries in the solution and soak them for about 5 minutes.
- Rinse the blueberries under cold water after soaking them with the vinegar solution.
- Dry the blueberries by laying them out on a clean kitchen towel or paper towels and patting them dry gently with another towel or paper towel.

Blueberry Smoothie

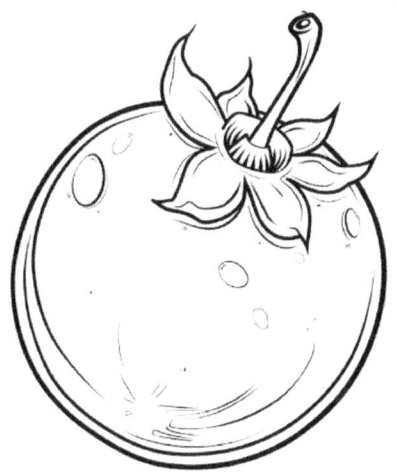

- 1 cup fresh or frozen blueberries
- 1 banana
- 1/2 cup Greek yogurt
- 1 cup milk (or almond milk)
- 1 tablespoon honey (optional)

1. Combine all ingredients in a blender.
2. Blend until smooth.
3. Pour into a glass and enjoy immediately.

Blueberry Pancakes

- 1 cup all-purpose flour
- 1 tablespoon sugar
- 1 teaspoon baking powder
- 1/2 teaspoon baking soda
- 1/4 teaspoon salt
- 1 cup buttermilk
- 1 egg
- 2 tablespoons melted butter
- 1 cup fresh or frozen blueberries

1. In a bowl, whisk together flour, sugar, baking powder, baking soda, and salt.
2. In another bowl, mix buttermilk, egg, and melted butter.
3. Pour wet ingredients into dry ingredients and stir until well combined.
4. Gently fold in the blueberries.
5. Heat a non-stick skillet over medium heat and lightly grease it.
6. Pour 1/4 cup of batter onto the skillet for each pancake.
7. Cook until bubbles form on the surface, then flip and cook until golden brown.
8. Serve with maple syrup.

Blueberry Yogurt Parfait

- 1 cup Greek yogurt
- 1/2 cup granola
- 1/2 cup fresh blueberries
- 1 tablespoon honey (optional)

1. In a glass or bowl, layer 1/2 cup Greek yogurt, followed by 1/4 cup granola and 1/4 cup blueberries.
2. Repeat the layers with the remaining ingredients.
3. Drizzle with honey if desired.
4. Enjoy within 1-3 days.

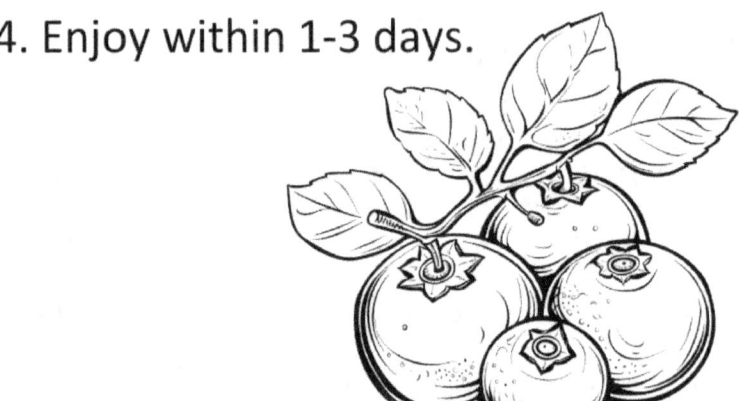

Vegan Blueberry Muffins

- 1 1/2 cups all-purpose flour
- 1/2 cup sugar
- 1/2 teaspoon salt
- 2 teaspoons baking powder
- 1/2 teaspoon baking soda
- 1/2 cup almond milk (or any plant-based milk)
- 1/3 cup vegetable oil
- 1 teaspoon vanilla extract
- 1 tablespoon apple cider vinegar
- 1 cup fresh or frozen blueberries

1. Preheat your oven to 375°F (190°C). Line a muffin tin with paper liners or lightly grease it.
2. In a large bowl, combine the flour, sugar, salt, baking powder, and baking soda. Mix well.
3. In another bowl, whisk together the almond milk, vegetable oil, vanilla extract, and apple cider vinegar.
4. Pour the wet ingredients into the dry ingredients and stir until well combined and smooth.
5. Gently fold in the blueberries.
6. Divide the batter evenly among the muffin cups, filling each about 2/3 full.
7. Bake for 20-25 minutes, or until a toothpick inserted into the center of a muffin comes out clean.
8. Allow the muffins to cool in the tin for about 5 minutes, then transfer them to a wire rack to cool completely.

Lemons

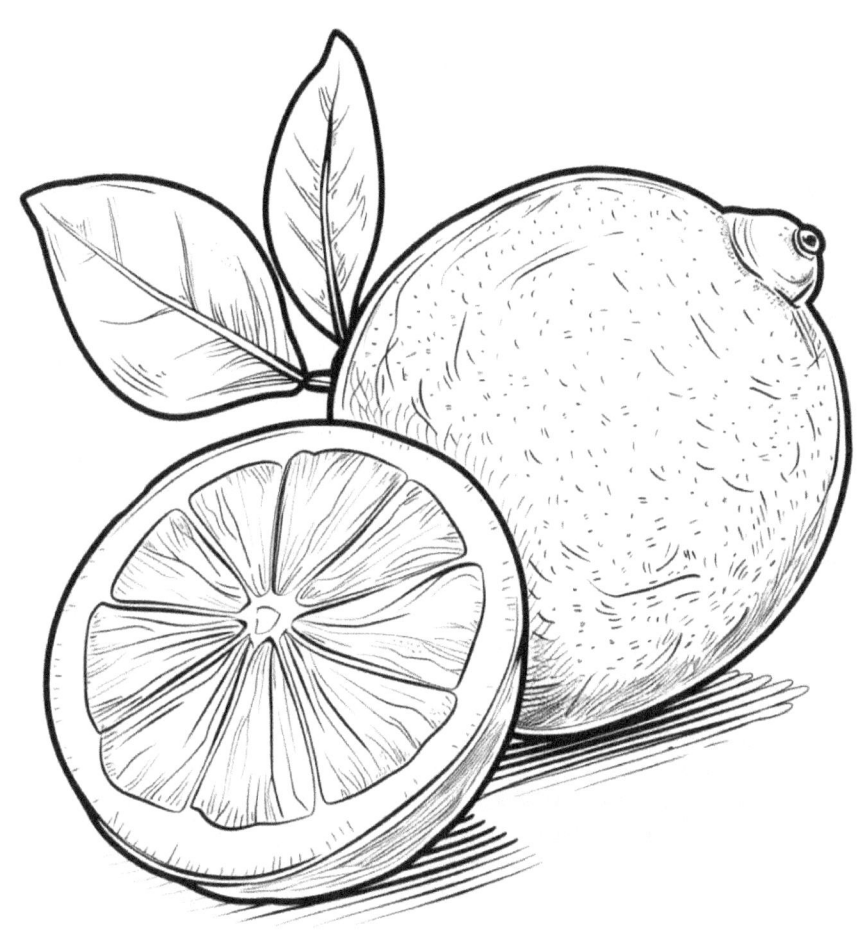

NUTRITION FACTS

Hydration
Adding lemon to water can make it more palatable, encouraging better hydration. Proper hydration is essential for overall health, including maintaining skin elasticity and supporting kidney function.

Skin Health
The antioxidants and vitamin C in lemons help combat skin damage caused by the sun and pollution, reduce wrinkles, and improve overall skin texture.

Alkalizes the Body
Despite their acidic taste, lemons have an alkalizing effect on the body when metabolized, which can help balance the body's pH levels.

Aids Digestion
The acidic nature of lemons can stimulate the production of digestive juices, improving digestion. Lemon juice can also help alleviate symptoms of indigestion, such as bloating and heartburn.

Kidney Stone Prevention
The citric acid in lemons may help prevent the formation of kidney stones by increasing urine volume and pH, creating a less favorable environment for stone formation.

Step-by-Step Cleaning Instructions

- Hold lemons under cold running water to remove any loose dirt or debris.
- Use a vegetable brush to scrub the lemons surface gently to remove any wax or pesticides. If you don't have a brush, a clean sponge can work as well.
- Soak lemons in a one-part vinegar three-part water solution for a few minutes to remove any remaining contaminants.
- After soaking, rinse the lemons thoroughly under cold water to wash away solution.
- Dry the lemons before storing them.

Classic Lemonade

- 1 cup fresh lemon juice (about 4-6 lemons)
- 1 cup granulated sugar
- 5 cups water
- Ice
- Lemon slices (for garnish)

Optional Ingredients for Extra Flavor:
- **Mint**
- **Strawberries or blueberries**
- **Slices or juice of oranges, limes, or grapefruits**
- **Pineapple**
- **Hibiscus**
- **Sparkling Water**
- **Ginger and Turmeric**

1. In a small saucepan, combine 1 cup of water and the sugar. Heat over medium heat, stirring until the sugar is dissolved to create a simple syrup. Allow to cool before the next step.
2. In a large pitcher, combine the lemon juice, simple syrup, and the remaining 4 cups of water. Stir well.
3. Serve over ice and garnish with lemon slices.

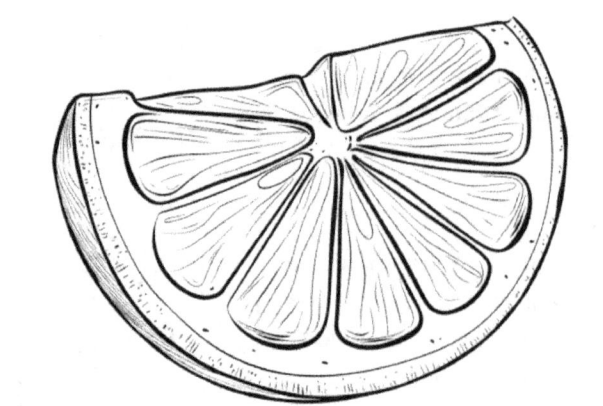

Lemon Bars

Ingredients for the crust:
- 1 cup unsalted butter, softened
- 1/2 cup granulated sugar
- 2 cups all-purpose flour
- 1/4 teaspoon salt

Ingredients for the filling:
- 4 large eggs
- 1 1/2 cups granulated sugar
- 1/4 cup all-purpose flour
- 2/3 cup fresh lemon juice
- Zest of 2 lemons

1. Preheat your oven to 350°F (175°C). Line a 9x13-inch baking pan with parchment paper.
2. In a bowl, stir together the butter and sugar for the crust. Mix in the flour and salt until the dough forms.
3. Press the dough evenly into the prepared pan. Bake for 15-20 minutes, or until lightly golden.
4. In another bowl, whisk together the eggs, sugar, flour, lemon juice, and lemon zest for the filling.
5. Pour the filling over the baked crust and return to the oven. Bake for an additional 20-25 minutes, or until the filling is set.
6. Allow to cool completely before cutting into squares. Dust with powdered sugar if desired.

Lemon Sorbet

- 1 cup water
- 1 cup granulated sugar
- 1 cup fresh lemon juice (about 4-5 lemons)
- 1 tablespoon lemon zest
- 1/2 cup cold water

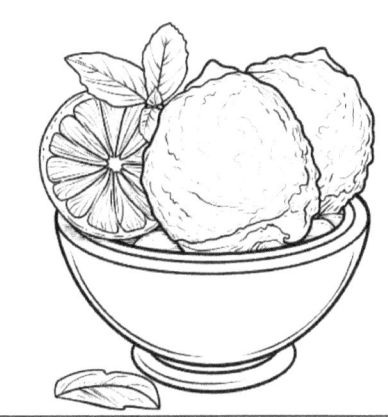

1. Make the Simple Syrup:
- In a medium saucepan, combine the water and sugar. Bring to a boil over medium heat, stirring until the sugar is dissolved.
- Remove from heat and let cool to room temperature.
2. Prepare the Sorbet Mixture:
- In a large bowl, combine the lemon juice, lemon zest, and cold water. Stir in the cooled simple syrup.
- Cover and refrigerate the mixture for at least 2 hours, or until thoroughly chilled.
3. Churn and Freeze:
- Pour the chilled mixture into an ice cream maker or blender and churn according to the manufacturer's instructions.
- Transfer the sorbet to an airtight container and freeze for at least 2 hours, or until firm.

Lemon Herb Salad Dressing

- 1/4 cup fresh lemon juice
- 1/2 cup olive oil
- 1 garlic clove, minced
- 1 teaspoon Dijon mustard
- 1 tablespoon honey
- 1 tablespoon chopped fresh herbs (such as parsley, basil, or thyme)
- Salt and pepper to taste

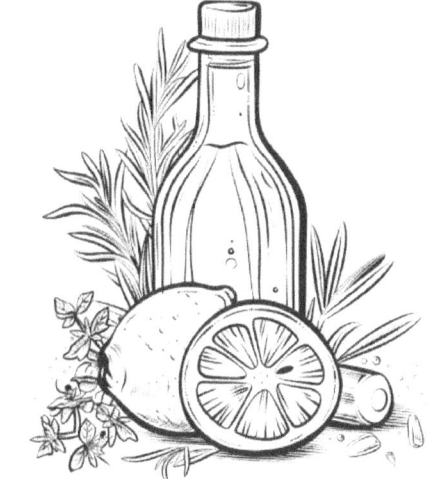

1. In a small bowl, whisk together the lemon juice, garlic, Dijon mustard, and honey.
2. Slowly add the olive oil while whisking continuously until the dressing is emulsified.
3. Stir in the fresh herbs and season with salt and pepper.
4. Use immediately or store in the refrigerator for up to one week.

Sweet Potatoes

NUTRITION FACTS

Macros in Sweet Potatoes:
- Calories: 112
- Protein: 2 grams
- Total Carbs: 26 grams
- Dietary Fiber: 0
- Sugars: 5 grams
- Total Fat: 0.1
- Cholesterol: 0

Vitamins in Sweet Potatoes:
- Vitamin A
- Vitamin C
- Vitamin B6
- Vitamin B1
- Vitamin B2
- Vitamin B3
- Vitamin B5
- Vitamin B9
- Vitamin E
- Vitamin K

Amino Acids in Sweet Potatoes:
- Tryptophan
- Threonine
- Isoleucine
- Leucine
- Lysine
- Methionine
- Phenylalanine
- Valine

Minerals in Sweet Potatoes:
- Manganese
- Potassium
- Copper
- Magnesium
- Phosphorus
- Iron
- Calcium
- Zinc
- Sodium

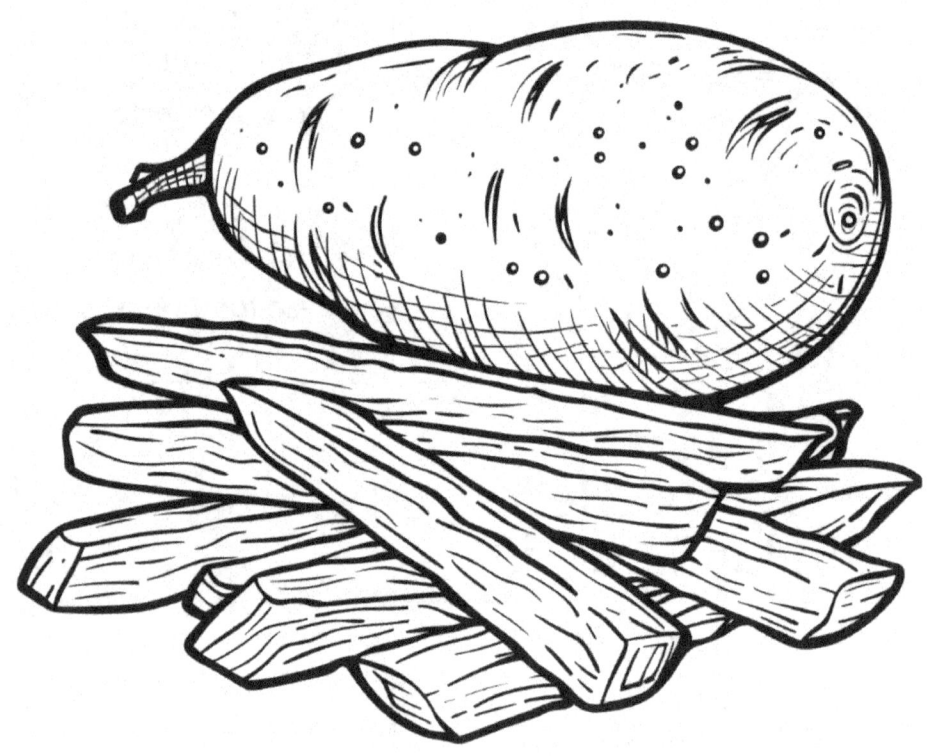

Step-by-Step Cleaning Instructions
- Hold sweet potato under cold running water while gently rubbing the surface, helping to loosen and remove dirt.
- Use a vegetable brush to scrub the skin of the sweet potato, focusing on the areas with visible dirt or blemishes. Make sure to scrub all sides of the sweet potato.
- After scrubbing, rinse the sweet potato under cold water to wash away any loosened dirt and debris.
- Inspect the sweet potato for any remaining dirt or blemishes. If necessary, scrub and rinse again.
- Pat the sweet potato dry with a clean kitchen towel or paper towel.
- Make sure sweet potato is completely dry before storing to prevent moisture buildup.

Mashed Sweet Potatoes

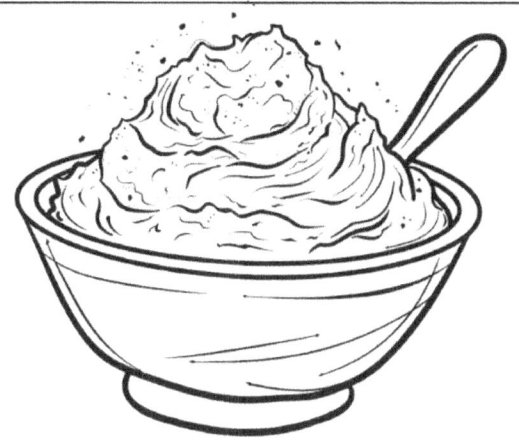

- 4 large sweet potatoes, peeled and cubed
- 1/4 cup milk or cream
- 2 tablespoons butter
- Salt and/or pepper to taste

1. Boil the sweet potatoes in a large pot of salted water until tender, about 15-20 minutes.
2. Drain and return the sweet potatoes to the pot.
3. Add milk, butter, salt, and pepper.
4. Mash and mix until smooth and creamy.

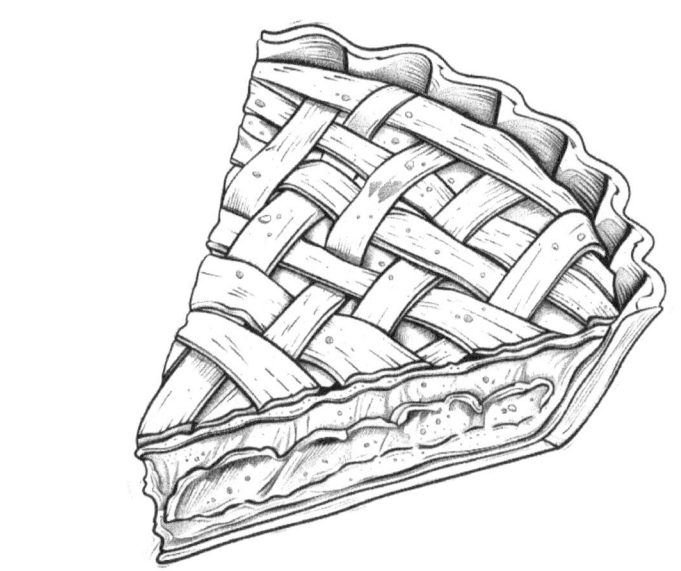

Sweet Potato Fries

- 2 large sweet potatoes, cut into thin fries
- 2 tablespoons olive oil
- Salt and pepper to taste
- Optional: paprika, chili powder, or cinnamon for extra flavor

1. Preheat your oven to 425°F (220°C).
2. In a bowl, toss the sweet potato fries with olive oil, salt, pepper, and any additional seasonings.
3. Spread the fries on a baking sheet in a single layer.
4. Bake for 20-25 minutes, flipping halfway through, until they are crispy and golden brown.

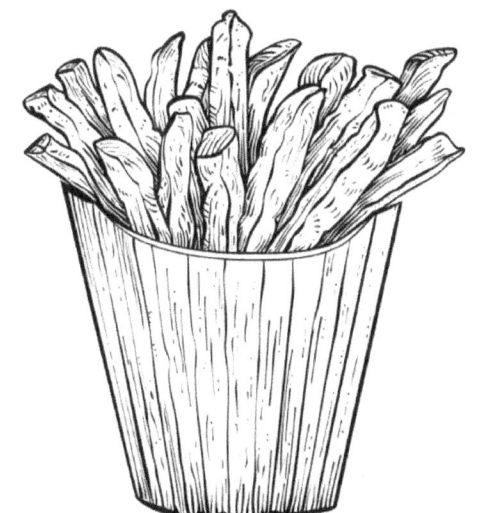

Roasted Sweet Potatoes

- 2 large sweet potatoes, peeled and cubed
- 2 tablespoons olive oil
- Salt and pepper to taste
- Optional: paprika, garlic powder, or rosemary for extra flavor

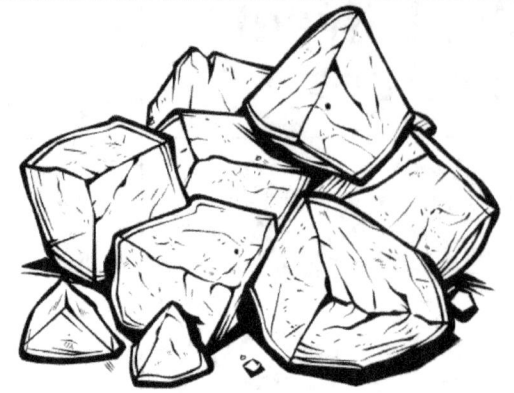

1. Preheat your oven to 400°F (200°C).
2. In a bowl, toss the sweet potato cubes with olive oil, salt, pepper, and any additional seasonings.
3. Spread the sweet potatoes on a baking sheet in a single layer.
4. Roast for 25-30 minutes, turning halfway through, until they are tender and slightly crispy.

Sweet Potato Soup

- 2 large sweet potatoes, peeled and cubed
- 1 onion, chopped
- 2 cloves garlic, minced
- 4 cups vegetable or chicken broth
- 1 tablespoon olive oil
- Salt and pepper to taste
- Optional: 1/2 teaspoon ground cumin or curry powder for extra flavor

1. In a large pot, heat the olive oil over medium heat.
2. Add the onion and garlic, and sauté until softened.
3. Add the sweet potatoes and broth, and bring to a boil.
4. Reduce heat and simmer until the sweet potatoes are tender, about 20 minutes.
5. Use an immersion blender or a regular blender to puree the soup until smooth.
6. Season with salt, pepper, and any additional spices.

Broccoli

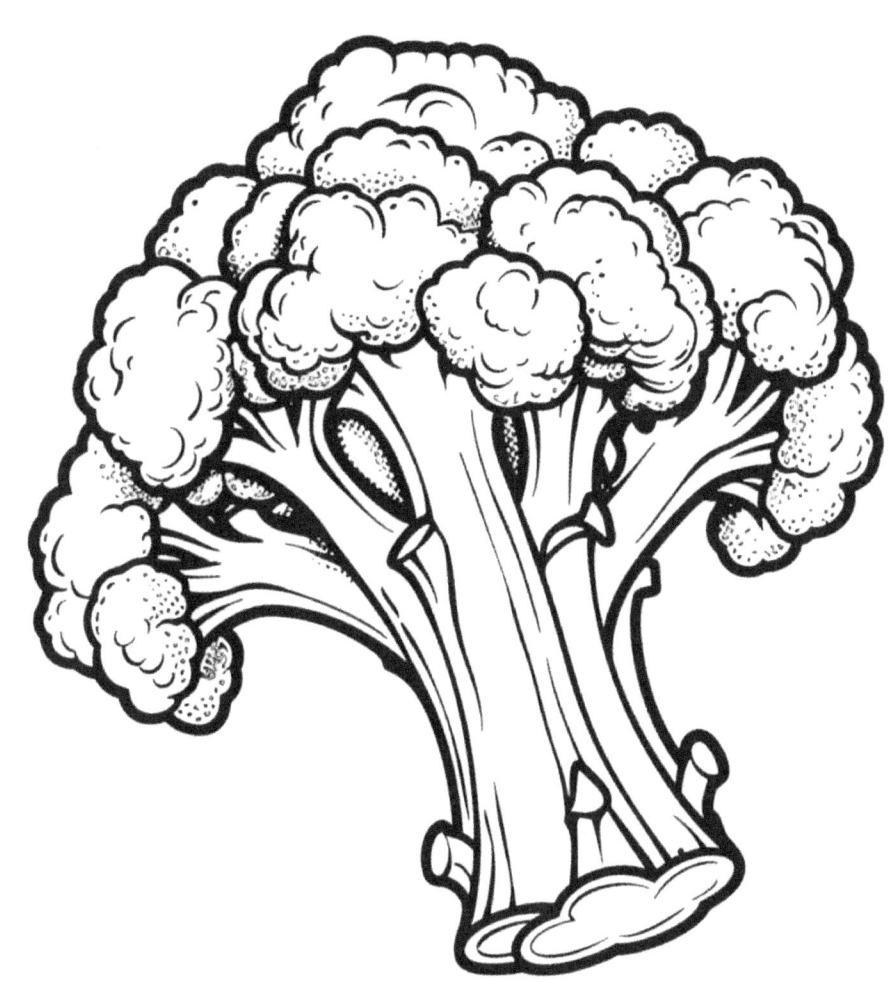

NUTRITION FACTS

Macros in 1 Cup of Broccoli:
- Calories: 31
- Total Fat: 0.3 grams
- Cholesterol: 0
- Sodium: 30 milligrams
- Total Carbs: 6 grams
- Dietary Fiber: 2.4 grams
- Sugars: 1.5 grams
- Protein: 2.6 grams

Vitamins and Minerals in 1 Cup of Broccoli:
- Vitamin A
- Vitamin C
- Vitamin K
- Folate
- Calcium
- Iron
- Potassium
- Magnesium
- Phosphorus

Anti-Aging Effects

The vitamin C and antioxidants in broccoli can reduce the damage caused by free radicals and promote healthy skin and tissues, contributing to a youthful appearance.

Cognitive Function

The choline and sulforaphane in broccoli can help aid in brain development and brain function.

Detoxification

The glucoraphanin, gluconasturtiin, and glucobrassicin found in broccoli helps to detox the body by removing harmful toxins.

Step-by-Step Cleaning Instructions

1. Remove damaged broccoli and cut into smaller florets.
2. Soak broccoli in a bowl of cold water with a few tablespoons of salt for 5-10 minutes. (Optional) Use a vegetable brush to scrub the stems and larger florets.
3. Rinse thoroughly under cold running water, rubbing the florets and stems with your fingers.
4. Drain broccoli in a colander and pat dry with a clean towel or paper towel. Let it air dry completely if storing.

Roasted Broccoli

- 1 head of broccoli, cut into florets
- 2 tablespoons olive oil
- Salt and pepper to taste
- Optional: garlic powder, lemon zest, or grated Parmesan cheese

1. Preheat your oven to 425°F (220°C).
2. Toss the broccoli florets with olive oil, salt, pepper, and any optional seasonings.
3. Spread the broccoli on a baking sheet in a single layer.
4. Roast for 20-25 minutes, stirring halfway through, until the edges are crisp and the broccoli is tender.
5. Sprinkle with Parmesan cheese or lemon zest before serving, if desired.

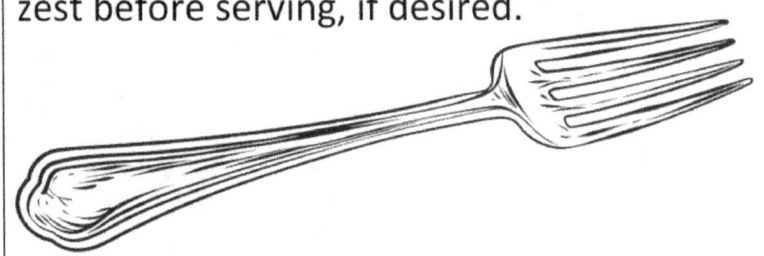

Broccoli Stir-Fry

- 1 head of broccoli, cut into florets
- 1 tablespoon vegetable oil
- 2 cloves garlic, minced
- 2 tablespoons soy sauce
- 1 tablespoon oyster sauce (optional)
- 1 teaspoon sesame oil
- Optional: sliced bell peppers, carrots, or other vegetables

1. Heat vegetable oil in a large skillet or wok over medium-high heat.
2. Add garlic and cook for about 30 seconds, until fragrant.
3. Add the broccoli (and any other vegetables) and stir-fry for 5-7 minutes, until the vegetables are tender-crisp.
4. Stir in soy sauce, oyster sauce, and sesame oil. Cook for another 1-2 minutes.
5. Serve hot over rice or noodles.

Broccoli and Cheese Stuffed Peppers

- 4 bell peppers
- 1 head broccoli, cut into florets
- 1 cup cooked quinoa
- 1 cup shredded cheddar cheese
- 1/2 cup diced onion
- 1/2 cup diced tomatoes
- 2 cloves garlic, minced
- 2 tbsp olive oil
- Salt and pepper to taste

1. Preheat the oven to 375°F (190°C).
2. Blanch the broccoli in boiling water for 3 minutes, then drain and chop finely.
3. In a large skillet, heat olive oil over medium heat. Add onion and garlic, and sauté until softened.
4. Stir in chopped broccoli, cooked quinoa, diced tomatoes, and cheddar cheese. Season with salt and pepper.
5. Cut the tops off the bell peppers and remove the seeds. Stuff the peppers with the broccoli mixture.
6. Place the stuffed peppers in a baking dish and bake for 25-30 minutes until the peppers are tender.

Broccoli and Cheddar-Baked Potatoes

- 4 large potatoes
- 1 head broccoli, cut into florets
- 1 cup shredded cheddar cheese
- 1/2 cup sour cream
- 1/4 cup milk
- 3 tbsp butter
- Salt and pepper to taste

1. Preheat the oven to 400°F (200°C).
2. Bake the potatoes for 1 hour or until tender.
3. Blanch the broccoli in boiling water for 3 minutes, then drain and chop finely.
4. Cut the potatoes in half and scoop out the flesh, leaving a thin shell.
5. In a bowl, mash the potato flesh with butter, sour cream, milk, salt, and pepper. Stir in the broccoli and cheddar cheese.
6. Spoon the mixture back into the potato shells and bake for 15-20 minutes until golden brown on top.

Avocado

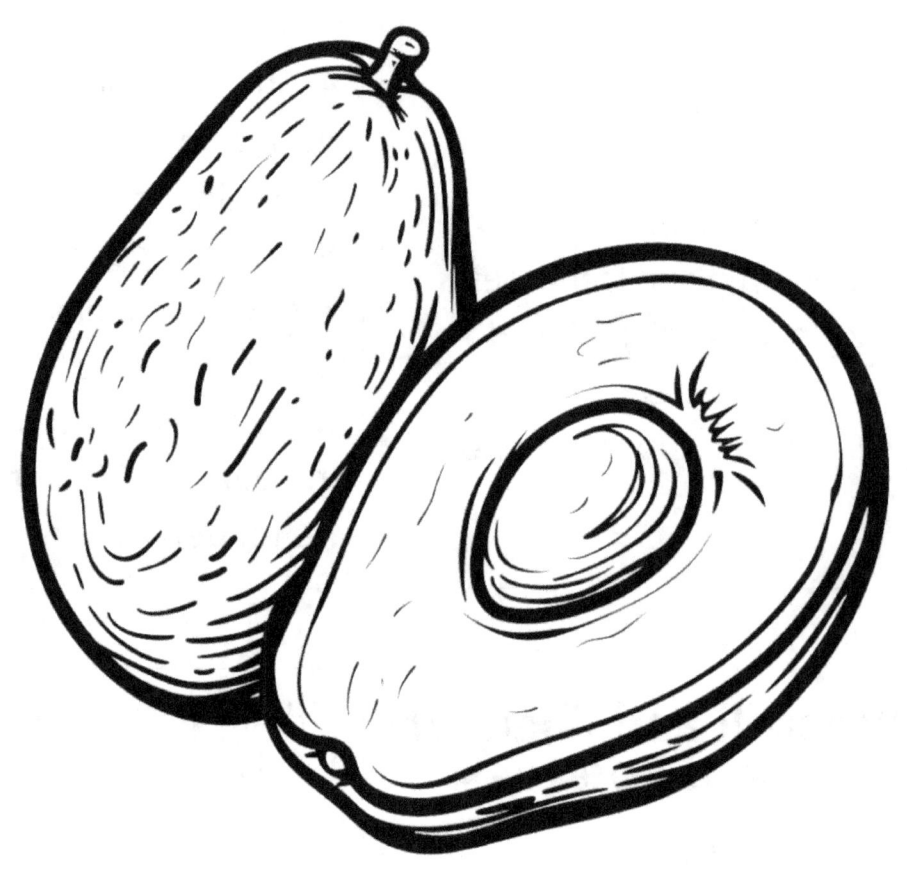

NUTRITION FACTS

Digestive Health
The fiber in avocados promotes a healthy gut microbiome by serving as a prebiotic, feeding beneficial bacteria.

Cancer Prevention
The high levels of antioxidants in avocados help protect cells from DNA damage, which can lead to cancer.

Heart Health
Potassium in avocados helps relax blood vessels, improving circulation and reducing strain on the heart.

Immune System Support
Avocados are nutrient rich containing Vitamins C, E, and B6, along with folate. They also help support the immune system by promoting the production and activity of white blood cells.

Brain Health
The antioxidants and healthy fats in avocados help protect the brain from oxidative damage and may reduce the risk of neurodegenerative diseases.

Metabolic Health
The B vitamins in avocados play a critical role in energy metabolism by helping convert food into energy.

Step-by-Step Cleaning Instructions

1. Rinse the Avocado under cold running water to remove surface dirt.
2. Use a soft brush or your hands to gently scrub the skin while rinsing.
3. Pat the avocado dry with a clean towel or paper towel.
4. Use a clean knife to cut the avocado in half. Twist to separate the halves, then remove the pit. Scoop out the flesh with a spoon.

Guacamole

- 2 ripe avocados
- 1 small onion, finely chopped
- 1-2 tomatoes, diced
- 1-2 cloves garlic, minced
- Juice of 1 lime
- Salt and pepper to taste
- Optional: chopped cilantro, diced jalapeño

1. Cut the avocados in half, remove the pits, and scoop the flesh into a bowl.
2. Mash the avocados with a fork until smooth or leave it slightly chunky, as you prefer.
3. Add the chopped onion, diced tomatoes, minced garlic, lime juice, salt, and pepper.
4. Mix well and add cilantro and jalapeño if desired.
5. Serve with tortilla chips or as a topping for tacos, salads, or sandwiches.

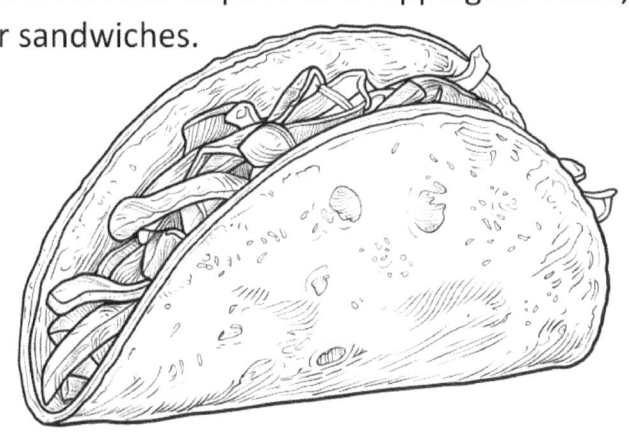

Avocado Toast

- 1 ripe avocado
- 2 slices of bread, toasted
- Salt and pepper to taste
- Optional toppings: sliced tomatoes, radishes, poached egg, red pepper flakes, olive oil, or lemon juice

1. Mash the avocado in a bowl and season with salt and pepper.
2. Spread the mashed avocado evenly on the toasted bread.
3. Add your favorite toppings and serve immediately.

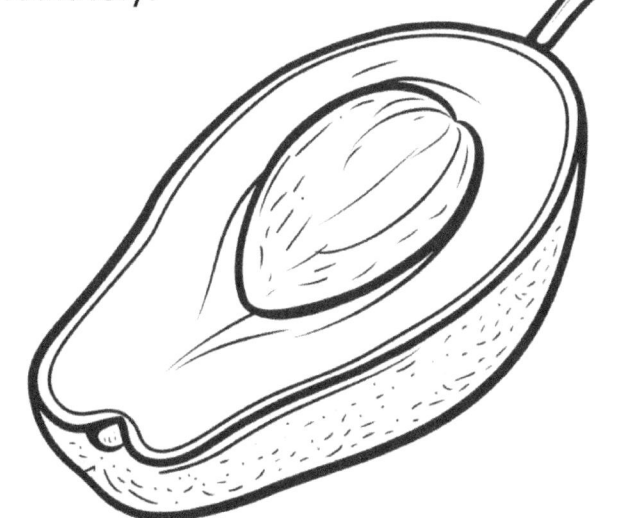

Avocado and Black Bean Tacos

- 2 ripe avocados, sliced
- 1 can black beans, rinsed and drained
- 1 cup corn kernels
- 1/2 cup diced red onion
- 1/4 cup chopped cilantro
- 1 lime, juiced
- 8 small corn tortillas
- Salt and pepper to taste

1. In a medium bowl, combine black beans, corn, red onion, cilantro, and lime juice. Season with salt and pepper.
2. Warm the tortillas in a skillet over medium heat.
3. Fill each tortilla with the avocado slices and black bean mixture.
4. Serve immediately.

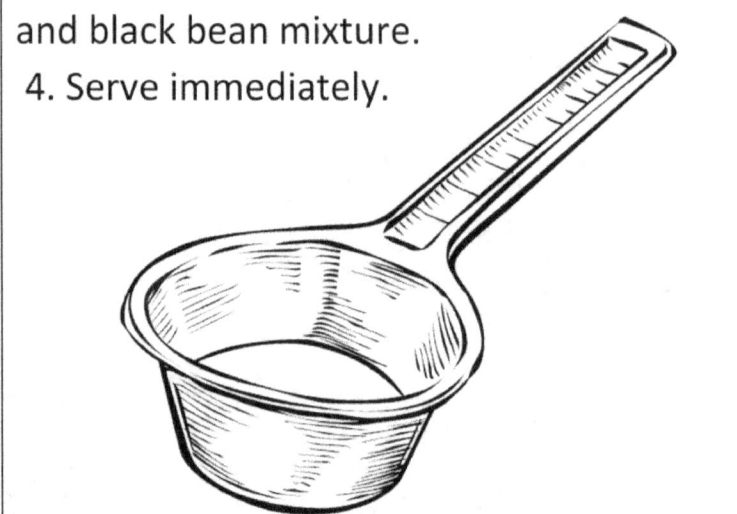

Avocado Sushi Rolls

- 1 cup sushi rice
- 2 cups water
- 2 tablespoons rice vinegar
- 1 tablespoon sugar
- 1/2 teaspoon salt
- 1 ripe avocado, sliced
- Nori sheets
- Soy sauce for serving

1. Rinse sushi rice until the water runs clear.
2. Combine rice and water in a pot and bring to a boil. Reduce heat to low and cook covered for 20 minutes or until rice is thoroughly cooked.
3. In a small bowl, mix rice vinegar, sugar, and salt. Stir into cooked rice.
4. Place a nori sheet on a bamboo sushi mat. Spread an even layer of rice over the nori, leaving a small border at the top.
5. Arrange avocado slices over the rice.
6. Roll the sushi tightly using the mat. Slice into pieces and serve with soy sauce.

Carrots

NUTRITION FACTS

Oral Health
Chewing raw carrots helps clean teeth and gums by removing plaque and food particles.

Weight Management
Carrots are low in calories, making them an excellent addition to a weight-loss diet. The fiber in carrots promotes feelings of fullness, reducing overall calorie intake.

Skin Health
Vitamins A and C in carrots help protect the skin from damage and promote healing. The high water content in carrots helps keep the skin hydrated and healthy.

Blood Sugar Regulation
Carrots help regulate blood sugar by slowing down the absorption of sugar into the bloodstream.

Cognitive Function
Carrots help protect the brain from oxidative stress and may reduce the risk of cognitive decline and neurodegenerative diseases.

Anti-Aging Effects
Carrots protect the skin from free radical damage, reducing signs of aging like wrinkles and fine lines. They also promote healthy skin and help to repair skin tissues.

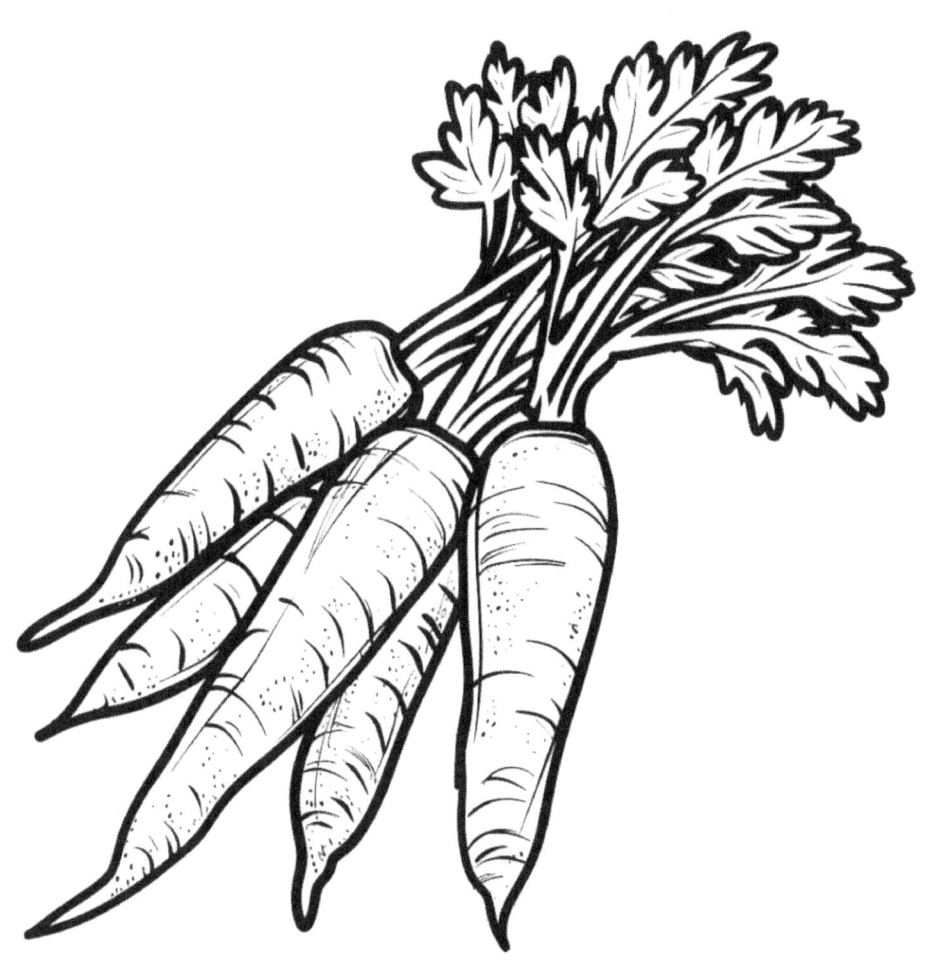

Step-by-Step Cleaning Instructions
1. Rinse the carrots under cold running water to remove surface dirt.
2. Use a vegetable brush to scrub the carrots thoroughly, focusing on any areas with visible dirt.
3. Cut off the tops and any thin, stringy roots at the bottom.
4. (Optional) Use a vegetable peeler to peel the carrots if desired. Not doing so retains the nutrients in the skin.
5. Give the carrots one last rinse under cold water to wash away any remaining debris.
6. Pat the carrots dry with a clean towel or paper towel if using them immediately. If storing, let them air dry completely.

Carrot and Pineapple Smoothie

- 2 large carrots, peeled and chopped
- 1 cup pineapple chunks
- 1 banana
- 1/2 cup coconut milk
- 1/2 cup pineapple juice

1. Place all ingredients in a blender.
2. Blend until smooth.
3. Pour into glasses and serve immediately.

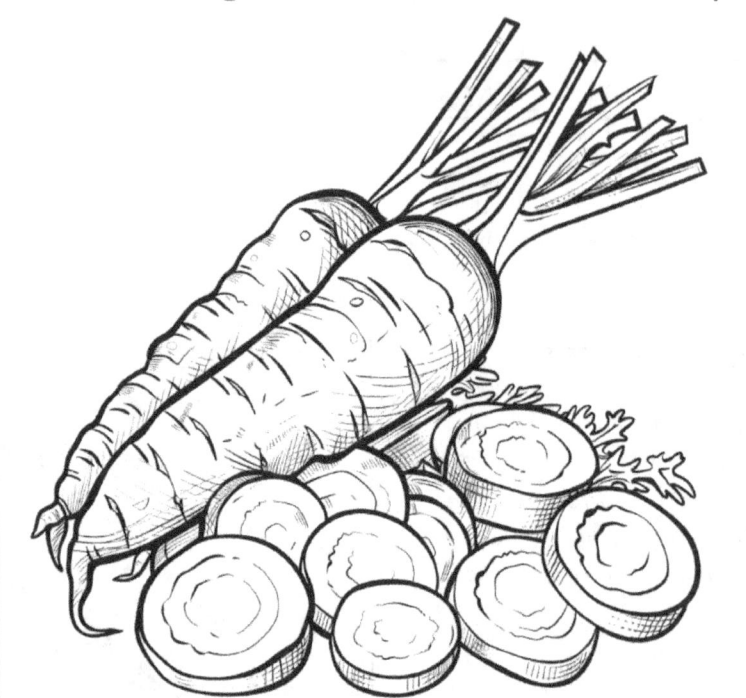

Carrot Cake

- 2 cups grated carrots
- 1 cup all-purpose flour
- 1 cup granulated sugar
- 1/2 cup vegetable oil
- 1/2 cup chopped walnuts or pecans (optional)
- 1/2 cup crushed pineapple, drained
- 2 eggs
- 1 teaspoon baking powder
- 1 teaspoon baking soda
- 1 teaspoon ground cinnamon
- 1/2 teaspoon salt
- Cream cheese frosting

1. Preheat oven to 350°F (175°C). Grease and flour a 9x13-inch baking pan.
2. In a large bowl, combine flour, sugar, baking powder, baking soda, cinnamon, and salt.
3. In another bowl, beat together oil and eggs. Stir in grated carrots, nuts (if using), and crushed pineapple.
4. Gradually add dry ingredients to the wet ingredients, stirring until well combined.
5. Pour batter into prepared pan and bake for 30-35 minutes, or until a toothpick inserted into the center comes out clean.
6. Allow cake to cool completely before topping with cream cheese frosting.

Roasted Carrots

- 1 pound carrots, peeled and sliced into sticks
- 2 tablespoons olive oil
- 1 teaspoon cumin
- 1/2 teaspoon paprika
- Salt and pepper to taste
- Fresh parsley, chopped (optional)

1. Preheat oven to 400°F (200°C).
2. In a bowl, toss carrots with olive oil, cumin, paprika, salt, and pepper until evenly coated.
3. Spread carrots in a single layer on a baking sheet.
4. Roast for 20-25 minutes, stirring halfway through, until carrots are tender and lightly caramelized.
5. Garnish with fresh parsley before serving.

Carrot Juice

- 4 large carrots
- 1 apple (optional)
- 1-inch piece of ginger (optional)
- One inch piece of turmeric
- One orange, peeled

1. Wash and peel the carrots.
2. Cut carrots (and apple and ginger, if using) into pieces that fit your juicer.
3. Juice the carrots and other ingredients.
4. Pour into a glass and serve immediately.
5. Alternative: Blend the ingredients in a blender and strain with a fine mesh strainer.

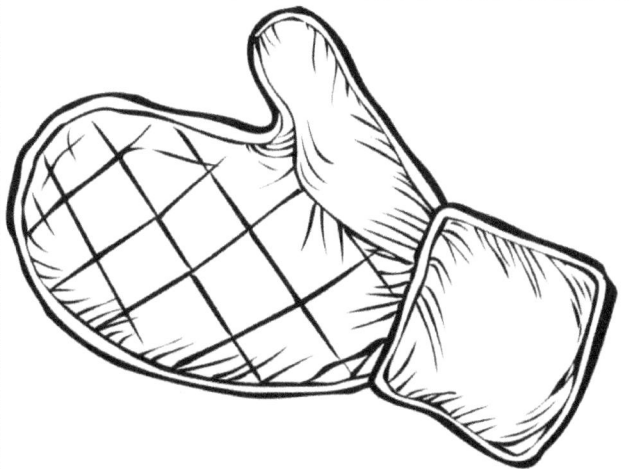

Apples

NUTRITION FACTS

Vitamins in Apples:
- **Vitamin A**
- **Vitamin C (Ascorbic Acid)**
- **Vitamin B1 (Thiamine)**
- **Vitamin B2 (Riboflavin)**
- **Vitamin B6 (Pyridoxine)**
- **Folate (Vitamin B9)**
- **Vitamin K1 (Phylloquinone)**
- **Vitamin E (Alpha-Tocopherol)**

Blood Health
Apples help cleanse the blood by eliminating toxins and promoting liver health.

Skin Benefits
The high vitamin C content helps reduce inflammation and promotes clear skin, reducing the risk of acne.

Enhanced Nutrition
The combination of vitamins, minerals, and fiber in apples can enhance the absorption of other nutrients from the diet, improving overall nutritional status.

Enhanced Energy/Performance
The 86% high water content and presence of potassium in apples help maintain electrolyte balance and hydration, enhancing physical performance.

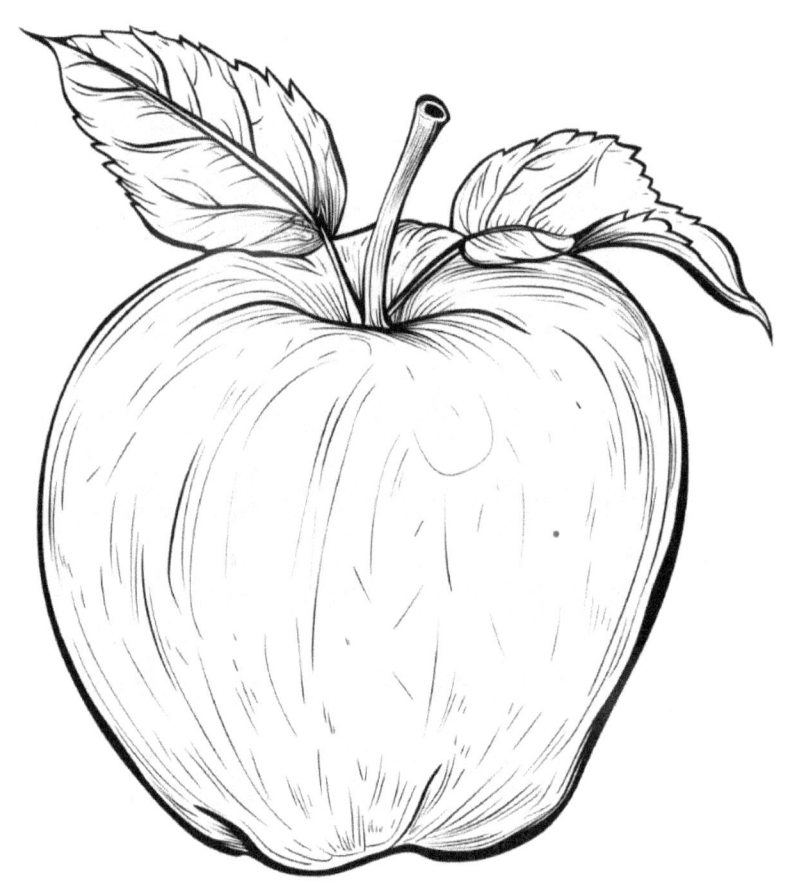

Step-by-Step Cleaning Instructions

1. Rinse the apple under cold running water to remove surface dirt.
2. Use a soft brush or your hands to gently scrub the apple's skin while rinsing.
3. (Optional) For extra cleaning, soak the apple in a mixture of water and white vinegar (1 part vinegar to 3 parts water) for a few minutes. This helps to remove pesticides and bacteria.
4. Rinse the apple thoroughly under cold running water to remove any vinegar residue.
5. Pat the apple dry with a clean towel or paper towel.

Fresh Apple Juice

- 6-8 medium-sized apples (choose a variety of sweet and tart apples for a balanced flavor)
- 1-2 tablespoons lemon juice (optional, to prevent oxidation)
- Sugar or honey to taste (optional)
- Water (if needed, to adjust consistency)

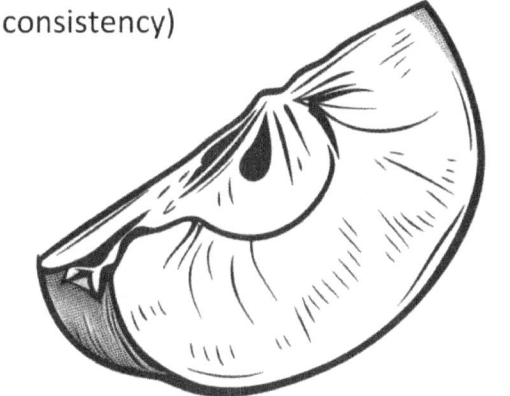

1. Wash the apples thoroughly under running water.
2. Core the apples and cut them into quarters. You can leave the skin on as it contains valuable nutrients.
3. Feed the apple quarters through your juicer, following the manufacturer's instructions and collect the juice in a clean container.
4. Alternatively, place the apple quarters in a blender. You may need to do this in batches depending on the size of your blender.
5. Blend the apples until smooth. You can add a small amount of water if the mixture is too thick.
6. Pour the blended apples through a fine mesh strainer or cheesecloth into a bowl. Use a spoon or spatula to press the pulp and extract as much juice as possible.
7. Taste the apple juice. If it's too tart, you can add a bit of sugar or honey to sweeten it.
8. If desired, add 1-2 tablespoons of lemon juice to enhance the flavor and prevent oxidation.
9. Pour the juice into glasses and serve immediately over ice, if desired.

Fresh apple juice can be stored in the refrigerator for up to 3 days. Shake well before serving as natural separation may occur.

Classic Apple Pie

- 6 cups thinly sliced apples
- 3/4 cup sugar
- 2 tablespoons all-purpose flour
- 1 teaspoon ground cinnamon
- 1/4 teaspoon ground nutmeg
- 1 tablespoon lemon juice
- 1 tablespoon butter
- Pastry for a double-crust 9-inch pie

1. Preheat oven to 425°F (220°C).
2. In a large bowl, mix apples, sugar, flour, cinnamon, nutmeg, and lemon juice.
3. Line a 9-inch pie pan with one pie crust. Fill with apple mixture and dot with butter.
4. Cover with top crust, seal edges, and cut several slits in the top to allow steam to escape.
5. Bake for 45-50 minutes or until crust is golden brown and apples are tender.

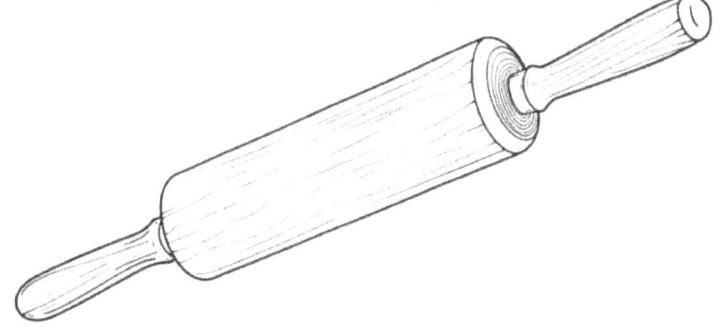

Homemade Apple Sauce

- 4 pounds of apples (about 8-10 medium apples), peeled, cored, and chopped
- 1 cup water
- 1/2 cup granulated sugar (optional, adjust to taste)
- 1 teaspoon ground cinnamon (optional)
- 1 tablespoon lemon juice (optional, to balance sweetness and preserve color)

1. Peel, core, and chop the apples into small chunks. For a smoother applesauce, chop the apples into smaller pieces.
2. In a large pot, combine the chopped apples, water, sugar, and cinnamon (if using). Bring the mixture to a boil over medium-high heat.
3. Reduce the heat to low, cover the pot, and simmer for about 20-30 minutes, or until the apples are very tender and easily mashed with a fork. Stir occasionally to prevent sticking.
4. For a chunky applesauce, use a potato masher or fork to mash the cooked apples to your desired consistency.
5. For a smoother applesauce, use an immersion blender directly in the pot or transfer the cooked apples to a blender or food processor and blend until smooth.
6. Taste the applesauce and adjust the sweetness by adding more sugar if needed. You can also add a bit of lemon juice to enhance the flavor and balance the sweetness.
7. If you like a spicier applesauce, you can add more cinnamon or even a pinch of nutmeg.
8. Allow the applesauce to cool to room temperature.
9. Transfer the applesauce to airtight containers and refrigerate for up to a week or freeze for longer storage.

Baked Apple Chips

- 2-3 apples, thinly sliced
- 1 teaspoon ground cinnamon
- 1 tablespoon sugar (optional)

1. Preheat the oven to 225°F (110°C). Line a baking sheet with parchment paper.
2. Arrange the apple slices in a single layer on the baking sheet.
3. Sprinkle with cinnamon and sugar if using.
4. Bake for 1.5 to 2 hours, flipping the apple slices halfway through, until they are dry and crisp.
5. Allow the apple chips to cool completely on a wire rack before serving.

Watermelon

NUTRITION FACTS

Hydration

Watermelon is about 90% water, making it an excellent choice for staying hydrated, especially during hot weather.

Antioxidants

Watermelon contains antioxidants like lycopene and beta-carotene, which help protect cells from damage and reduce inflammation.

Heart Health

Lycopene in watermelon may help reduce cholesterol levels and blood pressure, supporting cardiovascular health.

Digestive Health

The fiber content in watermelon aids in digestion and helps maintain a healthy gut.

Muscle Soreness Relief

Watermelon contains the amino acid citrulline, which has been linked to reduced muscle soreness and improved exercise performance.

Skin Health

The high-water content and vitamins in watermelon help keep the skin hydrated and may improve its appearance and elasticity.

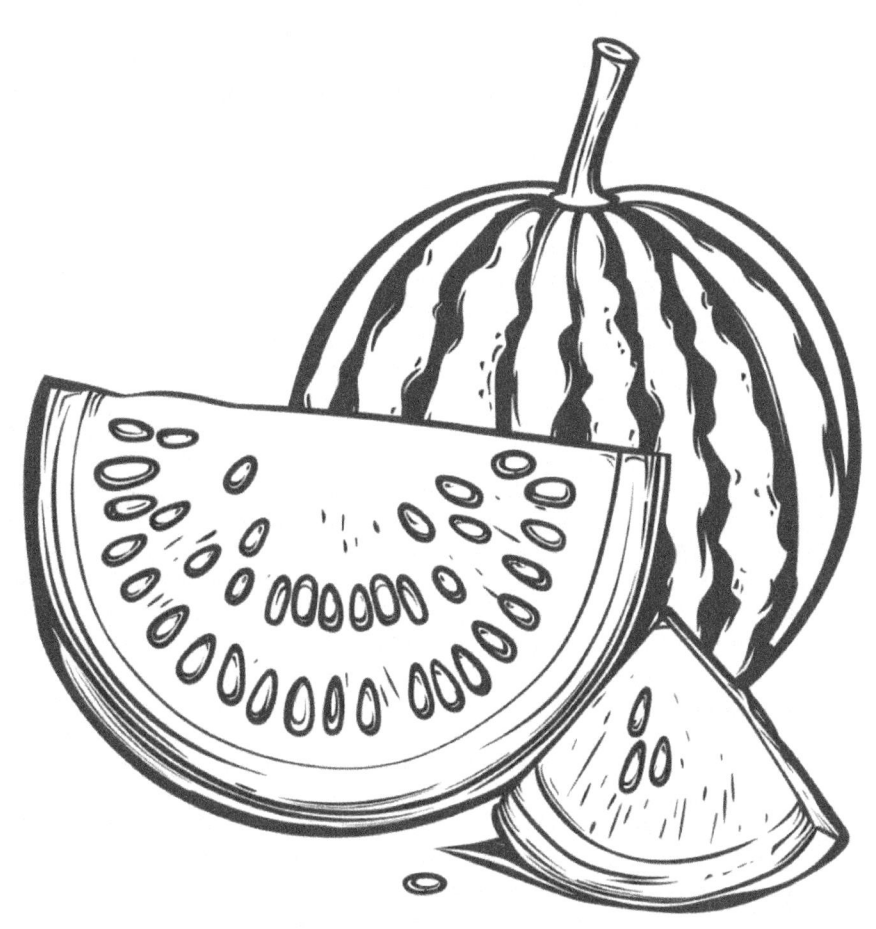

Step-by-Step Cleaning Instructions

- Rinse the entire watermelon under cold running water to remove any surface dirt.
- Use a clean vegetable brush to scrub the rind thoroughly while rinsing.
- Rinse the watermelon again under cold running water to wash away any loosened dirt.
- Pat the watermelon dry with a clean towel or paper towel.
- Use a clean knife and cutting board to cut the watermelon. Wash your hands before handling the flesh.

Watermelon Popsicles

- 4 cups cubed watermelon
- 1/4 cup lime juice
- 2 tablespoons honey (optional)

1. Blend the watermelon, lime juice, and honey until smooth.

2. Pour the mixture into popsicle molds.

3. Insert sticks and freeze for at least 4 hours or until solid.

4. Remove from molds and enjoy.

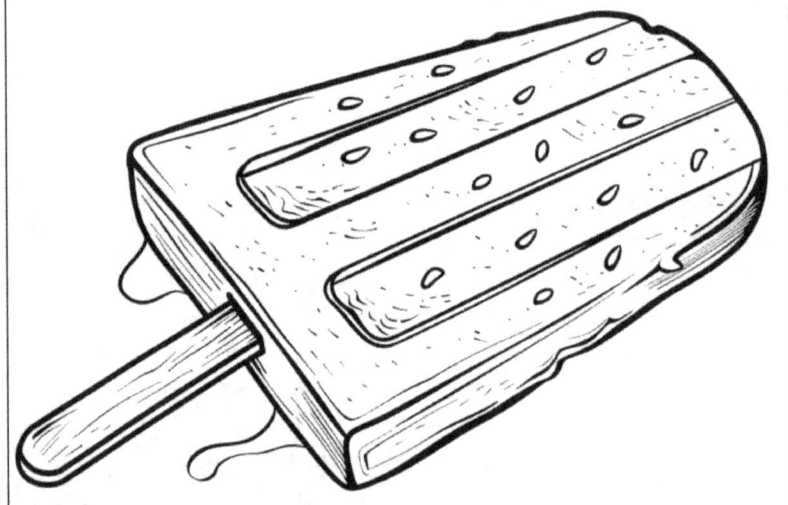

Watermelon Gazpacho

- 4 cups cubed watermelon
- 1 cucumber, peeled and chopped
- 1 red bell pepper, chopped
- 1/4 red onion, chopped
- 2 tablespoons olive oil
- 2 tablespoons red wine vinegar
- 1 tablespoon lime juice
- Salt and pepper to taste

1. In a blender, combine watermelon, cucumber, bell pepper, and red onion. Blend until smooth.

2. Add olive oil, red wine vinegar, lime juice, salt, and pepper. Blend again until well combined.

3. Chill in the refrigerator for at least 1 hour before serving.

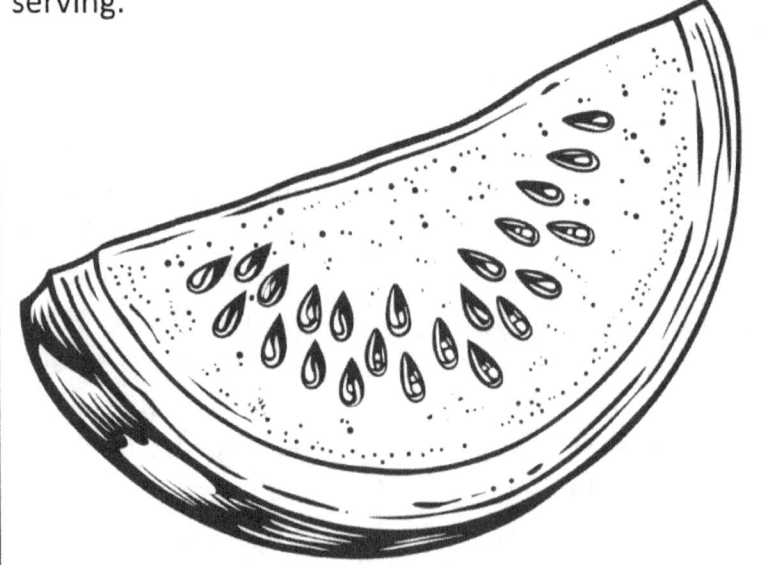

Watermelon Lemonade

- 4 cups cubed watermelon
- 1 cup freshly squeezed lemon juice (about 4-5 lemons)
- 1/2 cup granulated sugar (adjust to taste)
- 4 cups cold water
- Ice cubes
- Lemon slices and mint leaves for garnish (optional)

1. Cut the watermelon into cubes, removing any seeds if necessary.
2. In a blender, add the cubed watermelon and blend until smooth.
3. In a large pitcher, combine the freshly squeezed lemon juice and granulated sugar. Stir until the sugar is dissolved.
4. Pour the blended watermelon juice through a fine-mesh strainer into the pitcher with the lemon juice and sugar mixture. This will help remove any pulp or seeds from the watermelon juice.
5. Stir in the cold water until well combined. Taste and adjust sweetness if needed by adding more sugar, stirring until dissolved.
6. Refrigerate the lemonade for at least 1 hour to chill thoroughly. Serve over ice cubes in glasses.
7. Garnish each glass with a slice of lemon and a sprig of mint for a refreshing touch.

Watermelon Slushie

- 4 cups watermelon, cubed and frozen
- 1 tablespoon lime juice (about half a lime)
- 1 tablespoon honey or sugar (optional, adjust to taste)
- 1/2 cup water (adjust as needed)
- Fresh mint leaves for garnish (optional)

1. Cut a fresh watermelon into cubes and remove any seeds. Place the cubes on a baking sheet in a single layer and freeze them for at least 2-3 hours or until completely frozen.
2. Add the frozen watermelon cubes, lime juice, honey or sugar (if using), and water to a blender. Start with 1/2 cup of water and add more if needed to reach your desired consistency.
3. Blend the mixture until smooth and slushy. You may need to stop and stir the mixture a few times to ensure even blending.
4. Pour the watermelon slushie into glasses and garnish with fresh mint leaves if desired. Serve immediately for the best texture.

Cabbage

NUTRITION FACTS

Here are Some Ways to Elevate the Flavor and Texture of Cabbage:

- Sautéing
- Roasting
- Coleslaw
- Soups and Stews
- Stir-Fries
- Stuffed Cabbage
- Salads
- Grilled Cabbage

Rich in Nutrients
Cabbage is packed with essential vitamins and minerals, including vitamins C and K, folate, potassium, and calcium.

Boosts Immunity
The high vitamin C content in cabbage helps support a healthy immune system, aiding in the body's ability to fight off infections and illnesses.

Cancer Prevention
Cruciferous vegetables like cabbage contain compounds called glucosinolates, which have been studied for their potential to reduce the risk of certain types of cancer.

High in Fiber
The fiber content in cabbage supports digestive health, helps maintain regular bowel movements, and can aid in weight management by promoting a feeling of fullness.

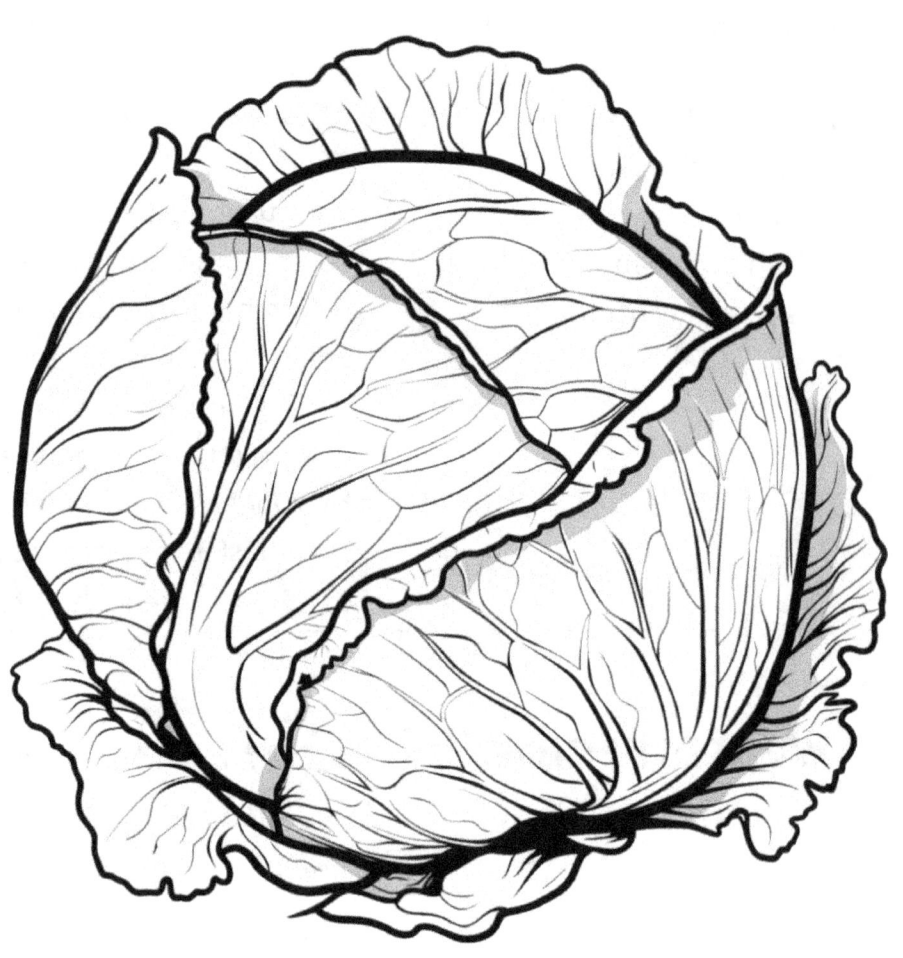

Step-by-Step Cleaning Instructions

- Remove and discard the outermost leaves of the cabbage, as they may be dirty or damaged.
- Rinse the cabbage head under cold running water to remove any loose dirt.
- Cut the cabbage into quarters or halves and then separate the leaves if desired. This makes it easier to clean between the layers.
- Soak the cabbage pieces in a bowl of cold water for a few minutes. Gently agitate the water to help loosen any dirt or debris.
- After soaking, rinse each leaf or section under cold running water to ensure all dirt and debris are removed.
- Shake off excess water and pat the cabbage dry with a clean towel or paper towel. If storing, let the cabbage air dry completely.

Sautéed Cabbage

- 1 medium head of cabbage, thinly sliced
- 2 tablespoons olive oil
- 1 onion, thinly sliced
- 2 garlic cloves, minced
- Salt and pepper to taste
- 1 tablespoon apple cider vinegar (optional)

1. Heat olive oil in a large skillet over medium heat. Add onion and garlic, and sauté until softened.
2. Add cabbage and cook, stirring frequently, until cabbage is tender and slightly browned, about 10-15 minutes.
3. Season with salt and pepper. If using, stir in apple cider vinegar for a tangy flavor.
4. Serve hot.

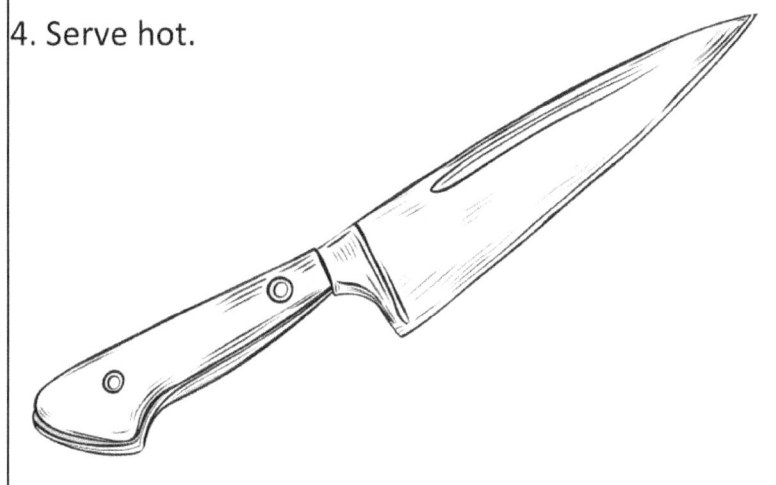

Stuffed Cabbage Rolls

- 1 large head of cabbage
- 1 pound ground beef or ground turkey meat
- 1 cup cooked rice
- 1 onion, finely chopped
- 1 egg, beaten
- 2 cups tomato sauce
- 1/2 cup beef or vegetable broth
- Salt and pepper to taste

1. Preheat oven to 350°F (175°C).
2. Bring a large pot of water to a boil. Carefully peel off 12 large cabbage leaves and blanch them in boiling water for 2 minutes. Remove and drain.
3. In a bowl, mix ground beef, rice, onion, egg, salt, and pepper.
4. Place a spoonful of meat mixture in the center of each cabbage leaf. Fold in the sides and roll up.
5. Place rolls seam-side down in a baking dish. Pour tomato sauce and broth over the rolls.
6. Cover with foil and bake for 1 hour, or until cabbage is tender and filling is cooked thoroughly.

Classic Coleslaw

- 1 medium head of cabbage, shredded
- 2 large carrots, grated
- 1 cup mayonnaise
- 1/4 cup apple cider vinegar
- 2 tablespoons sugar
- Salt and pepper to taste

1. In a large bowl, combine shredded cabbage and grated carrots.
2. In a separate bowl, whisk together mayonnaise, vinegar, sugar, salt, and pepper.
3. Pour dressing over the cabbage mixture and toss to coat.
4. Chill in the refrigerator for at least an hour before serving.

Southern Cabbage with Sausage

- 1 head green cabbage, chopped
- 1 lb smoked sausage, sliced
- 1 onion, chopped
- 2 cloves garlic, minced
- 1 cup chicken broth
- Salt and pepper to taste

1. In a large skillet, cook sausage over medium heat until browned. Remove and set aside.
2. Add onion to the skillet and sauté until translucent.
3. Add garlic and cook for another minute.
4. Stir in cabbage and cook until wilted, about 10 minutes.
5. Pour in chicken broth and cook for another 10 minutes until cabbage is tender.
6. Return sausage to the skillet, season with salt and pepper, and cook until heated through.

Tomatoes

NUTRITION FACTS

Ways Tomatoes Can Enhance Dish Taste:

- Umami Flavor
- Natural Sweetness
- Versatility
- Aromatic
- Color
- Moisture Content
- Nutrient Synergy
- Caramelization
- Flavor Absorption

Improved Sleep Quality

Compounds in tomatoes can help regulate melatonin levels, promoting better sleep patterns.

Mental Health

Folate in tomatoes helps in the synthesis of neurotransmitters like serotonin and dopamine, which regulate mood and reduce the risk of depression.

Nutrition Absorption

The natural acids in tomatoes can enhance the bioavailability of nutrients, improving the absorption of essential vitamins and minerals from other foods consumed with tomatoes.

Oral Health

The acidic nature of tomatoes acts as a natural astringent, helping to clean teeth and reduce plaque buildup.

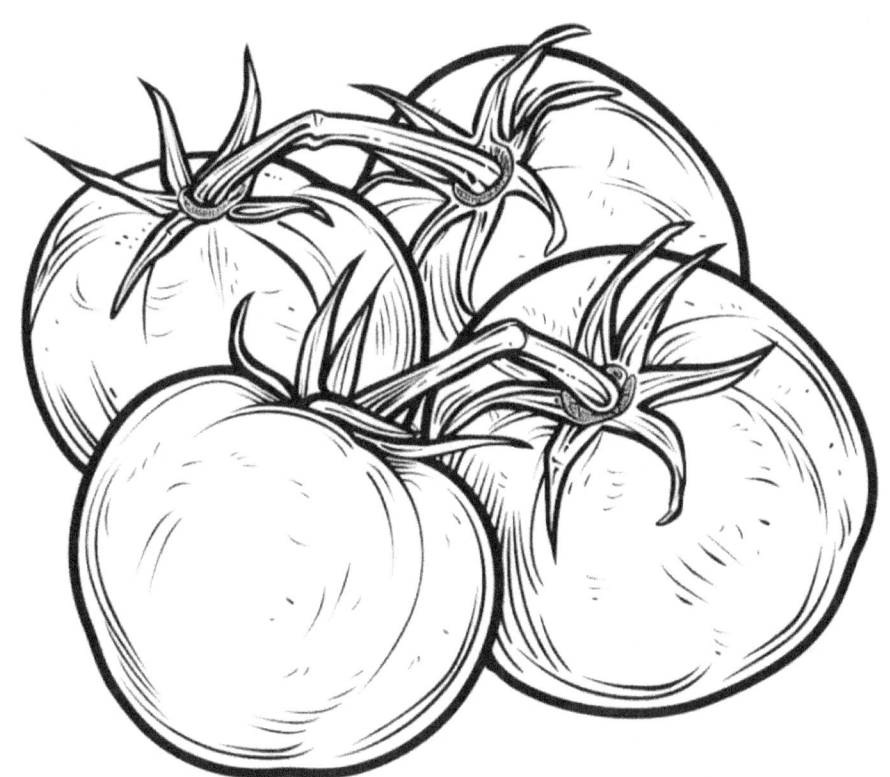

Step-by-Step Cleaning Instructions

- Rinse the tomatoes under cold running water to remove surface dirt.
- Use your hands or a soft vegetable brush to gently scrub the tomatoes' skin while rinsing. Be careful not to damage the skin.
- (Optional)For extra cleaning, soak the tomatoes in a mixture of water and white vinegar (1 part vinegar to 3 parts water) for a few minutes. This helps to remove pesticides and bacteria.
- Rinse the tomatoes thoroughly under cold running water to remove any vinegar residue.
- Pat the tomatoes dry with a clean towel or paper towel.

Caprese Salad

- Fresh tomatoes, sliced
- Fresh mozzarella, sliced
- Fresh basil leaves
- Extra virgin olive oil
- Balsamic vinegar
- Salt and pepper

1. Arrange tomato slices and mozzarella slices on a plate, alternating between the two.
2. Tuck basil leaves between the slices.
3. Drizzle with olive oil and balsamic vinegar.
4. Season with salt and pepper to taste.

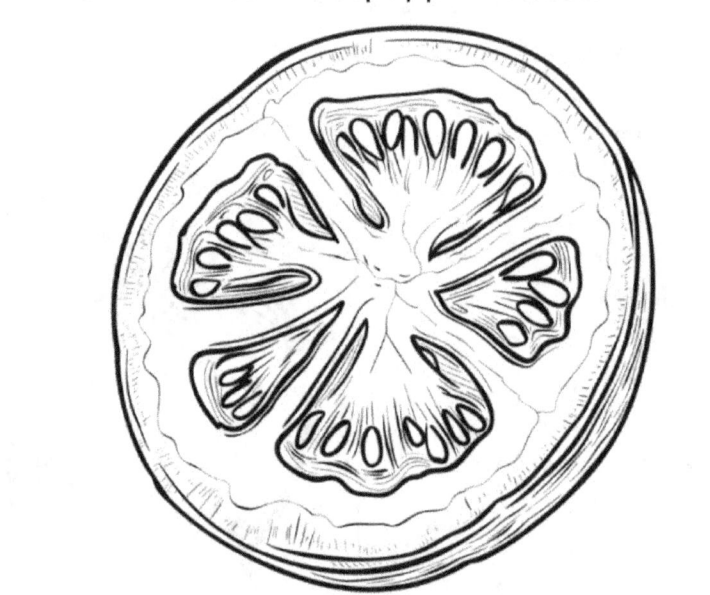

Spaghetti with Tomato Sauce

- 2 tablespoons olive oil
- 1 onion, chopped
- 2 garlic cloves, minced
- 5-6 ripe tomatoes, chopped
- 1 tablespoon tomato paste
- 1 teaspoon sugar (optional)
- Salt and pepper to taste
- Fresh basil or parsley, chopped
- Spaghetti, cooked according to package instructions

1. Heat olive oil in a pan over medium heat. Add onion and garlic, and sauté until soft.
2. Add chopped tomatoes, tomato paste, and sugar if using. Simmer for 15-20 minutes.
3. Season with salt, pepper, and fresh herbs.
4. Toss the sauce with cooked spaghetti and serve.

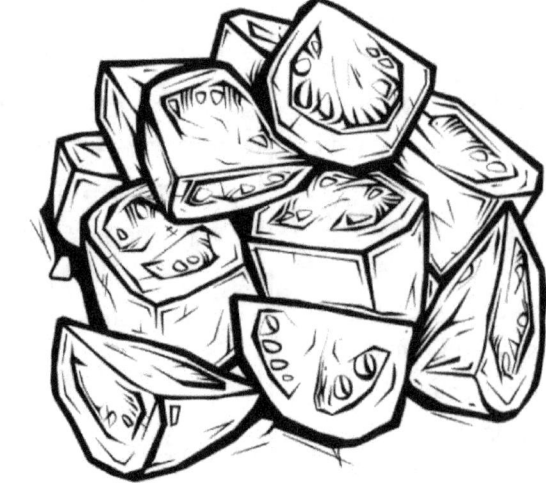

Homemade Salsa

- 4 ripe tomatoes, diced
- 1 small red onion, finely chopped
- 1-2 jalapeño peppers, seeded and finely chopped
- 1/4 cup fresh cilantro, chopped
- Juice of 1 lime
- 1-2 garlic cloves, minced
- Salt and pepper to taste

1. In a medium bowl, combine the diced tomatoes, red onion, jalapeño peppers, cilantro, and garlic.
2. Squeeze the lime juice over the mixture.
3. Add salt and pepper to taste.
4. Mix everything together until well combined or use a food processor to chop finely.
5. Let the salsa sit for about 15-30 minutes to allow the flavors to meld.
6. Serve with tortilla chips, tacos, grilled meats, or any other favorite dishes.

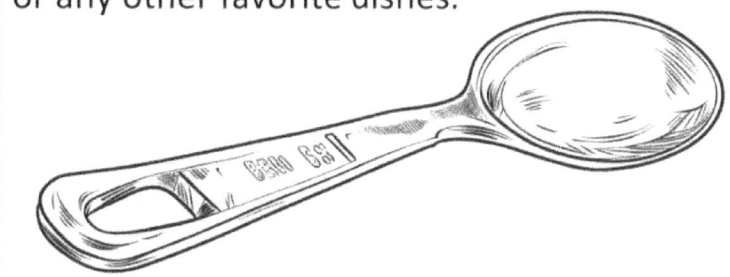

Homemade Ketchup

- 1 can (15 oz) of tomato sauce
- 1/4 cup of apple cider vinegar
- 1/4 cup of brown sugar
- 1 teaspoon of garlic powder
- 1 teaspoon of onion powder
- 1/2 teaspoon of salt

1. In a medium saucepan, combine the tomato sauce, apple cider vinegar, brown sugar, garlic powder, onion powder, and salt. Stir until smooth.
2. Place the saucepan over medium heat. Bring the mixture to a simmer, then reduce the heat to low.
3. Let the mixture simmer for about 20-25 minutes, stirring occasionally to prevent sticking. The ketchup will thicken as it cooks.
4. Once the ketchup has reached your desired consistency, remove it from the heat and let it cool. Transfer the ketchup to a jar or airtight container and store it in the refrigerator.

Mushrooms

NUTRITION FACTS

Nutrient Dense
Mushrooms provide essential nutrients, including vitamins, minerals, and antioxidants, while being low in calories.

Dietary Fiber
They are a good source of dietary fiber, which promotes healthy digestion and can help maintain stable blood sugar levels.

Support for Mental Health
Mushrooms certain compounds that may support cognitive function and mental health.

Rich in Antioxidants
Mushrooms contain powerful antioxidants that help protect the body from oxidative stress and inflammation.

Versatility
Mushrooms can be used in a wide variety of dishes, from soups and salads to stir-fries and sauces, adding flavor and texture to meals.

Flavor Enhancement
Mushrooms have a unique umami flavor that can enhance the taste of dishes, reducing the need for added salt or fat.

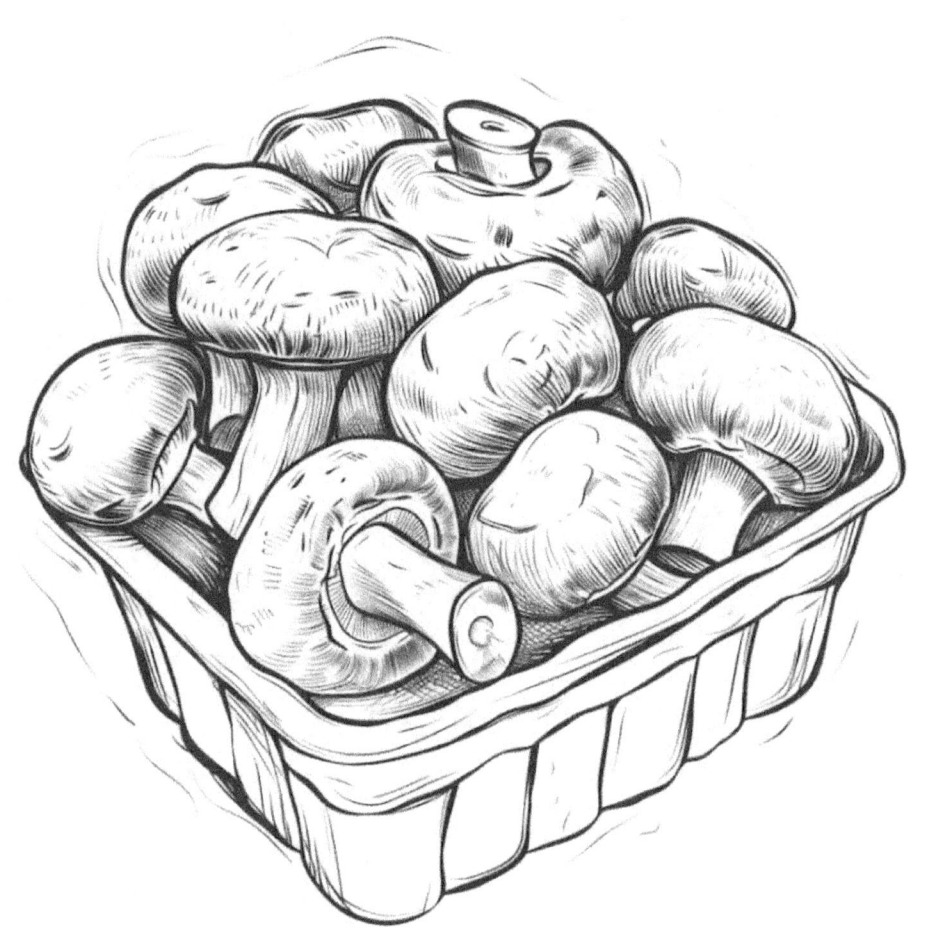

Step-by-Step Cleaning Instructions

- Inspect the mushrooms and remove any that are bruised or slimy.
- Use a soft brush or a dry paper towel to gently brush off any visible dirt from the mushrooms. Avoid using too much pressure to prevent damage.
- If the mushrooms are very dirty, you can quickly rinse them under cold running water. However, do this just before using them, as mushrooms absorb water and can become soggy.
- Pat the mushrooms dry with a clean towel or paper towel immediately after rinsing. Make sure they are completely dry before cooking or storing.
- Use a knife to trim the ends of the stems if they appear tough or dirty.

Mushroom Risotto

- 2 tablespoons olive oil
- 1 onion, chopped
- 2 garlic cloves, minced
- 1 1/2 cups Arborio rice
- 1/2 cup dry white wine
- 4 cups vegetable broth, kept warm
- 1 pound (450 grams) mushrooms, sliced
- 1/2 cup grated Parmesan cheese
- 2 tablespoons butter
- Salt and pepper to taste
- Fresh parsley, chopped (for garnish)

1. In a large skillet, heat olive oil over medium heat. Add the onion and garlic, and cook until soft.
2. Add the mushrooms and cook until they release their moisture and become golden brown. Remove from skillet and set aside.
3. In the same skillet, add the Arborio rice and cook, stirring constantly, for 1-2 minutes until lightly toasted.
4. Pour in the white wine and cook until evaporated.
5. Begin adding the warm vegetable broth, one ladle at a time, stirring frequently and waiting until the liquid is absorbed before adding more.
6. After about 20 minutes, when the rice is creamy and tender, stir in the cooked mushrooms, Parmesan cheese, and butter.
7. Season with salt and pepper, and garnish with fresh parsley.

Mushroom and Spinach Frittata

- 1 tablespoon olive oil
- 1/2 onion, chopped
- 2 garlic cloves, minced
- 1/2 pound (225 grams) mushrooms, sliced
- 2 cups fresh spinach
- 6 large eggs
- 1/4 cup milk
- 1/4 cup grated Parmesan cheese
- Salt and pepper to taste

1. Preheat oven to 375°F (190°C).
2. In an ovenproof skillet, heat the olive oil over medium heat. Add the onion and garlic, and cook until soft.
3. Add the mushrooms and cook until they release their moisture and become golden brown.
4. Add the spinach and cook until wilted.
5. In a bowl, whisk together the eggs, milk, Parmesan cheese, salt, and pepper.
6. Pour the egg mixture into the skillet and stir to combine with the vegetables.
7. Cook for a few minutes until the edges begin to set, then transfer the skillet to the oven.
8. Bake for 10-12 minutes, or until the frittata is set and golden brown on top.

Oyster Mushroom Tenders

- 10-12 large oyster mushrooms, cleaned and separated
- 1 cup all-purpose flour (or a gluten-free alternative)
- 1 cup non-dairy milk (such as almond, soy, or oat)
- 1 tablespoon apple cider vinegar (or lemon juice)
- 1 cup breadcrumbs (use gluten-free if needed)
- 1 teaspoon garlic powder, onion powder, and smoked paprika
- 1/2 teaspoon dried thyme, dried oregano, salt, and black pepper
- Oil for frying (such as vegetable or avocado oil)

1. In a bowl, combine the non-dairy milk and apple cider vinegar (or lemon juice). Let it sit for about 5 minutes to create a vegan buttermilk.
2. In a separate bowl, mix the flour with garlic powder, onion powder, smoked paprika, dried thyme, dried oregano, salt, and black pepper.
3. Place the breadcrumbs in a third bowl.
4. Dip and thoroughly coat each oyster mushroom in the flour mixture, shaking off any excess. Then dip it into the vegan buttermilk, and finally coat it with the breadcrumbs. Make sure the mushrooms are well-coated at each step.
5. In a large skillet, heat about 1/2 inch of oil over medium-high heat until hot (about 350°F or 175°C).
6. Fry the coated mushrooms in batches, being careful not to overcrowd the pan. Cook each side for about 3-4 minutes, or until golden brown and crispy. Transfer to a paper towel-lined plate to drain any excess oil.
7. Serve the vegan tenders hot with your favorite dipping sauces, such as vegan ranch, barbecue sauce, or ketchup.

Lion's Mane Steak

- 1 pound Lion's Mane mushrooms, cleaned and sliced into thick slabs
- 2 tablespoons olive oil
- 2 tablespoons soy sauce or tamari
- 2 tablespoons balsamic vinegar
- 1 tablespoon maple syrup or agave nectar
- 1 teaspoon smoked paprika
- 1 teaspoon garlic powder
- 1 teaspoon onion powder
- Salt and pepper to taste
- Fresh parsley for garnish (optional)

1. In a small bowl, mix together the soy sauce or tamari, balsamic vinegar, maple syrup or agave nectar, smoked paprika, garlic powder, and onion powder.
2. Place the mushroom slabs in a shallow dish or a resealable plastic bag. Pour the marinade over the mushrooms, ensuring they are well-coated. Let them marinate for at least 30 minutes, or up to 2 hours for more flavor.
3. In a large skillet, heat the olive oil over medium-high heat.
4. Remove the mushroom slabs from the marinade, letting any excess marinade drip off. Reserve the marinade. Place the mushrooms in the skillet and cook for about 4-5 minutes on each side, or until they are golden brown and crispy on the edges.
5. Pour the reserved marinade into the skillet and cook for an additional 1-2 minutes, until the sauce has reduced slightly and coats the mushrooms.
6. Season with salt and pepper to taste.
7. Transfer the mushroom steaks to a serving plate and garnish with fresh parsley if desired. Serve hot, with your favorite sides.

Substitutions

Sugar	Honey	Agave	Brown Sugar	Maple Syrup
Vegetable Oil/Butter	Avocado oil	Olive Oil	Coconut Oil	Flaxseed Oil
Milk	Almond Milk	Coconut Milk	Oat Milk	Soy Milk
Table Salt	Pink Himalayan Salt	Celtic Sea Salt	Kosher Salt	Lemon Juice
Chicken Broth	Vegetable Broth	Bouillon Cube	Water	Mushroom Broth
Eggs	Bananas	Flax Seed	Dates	Apple Sauce/Purée
All Purpose Flour	Almond Flour	(Whole) Wheat Flour	Coconut Flour	Self-Rising Flour